FUNDAMENTALS OF INFECTION CONTROL

An In-Service Orientation Program

Charles P. Craig, M.D.
Editor and Principal Author

D1384400

Medical Economics Books
Oradell, New Jersey 07649

Library of Congress Cataloging in Publication Data

Craig, Charles P.
Fundamentals of infection control.

Includes index.
1. Communicable diseases—Nursing. 2. Nosocomial
infections—Prevention. 3. Asepsis and antisepsis.
I. Title. [DNLM: 1. Cross infection—Prevention and
control. 2. Inservice training. WX 167 C886f]
RT95.C7 1983   616.9'045   81-81306
ISBN 0-87489-187-6

Cover design by James M. Walsh

ISBN 0-87489-187-6

Medical Economics Company Inc.
Oradell, New Jersey 07649

Printed in the United States of America

Contents

Publisher's notes

This versatile book has been written and designed to serve a dual purpose: For hospital staff instructors, it functions as a teaching resource for inservice education programs in hospital infection control. For the students in such programs, it functions both as a basic introductory reference and self-review.

Charles P. Craig, M.D., presents the study material in clearly written text form—the 12 chapters that make up the first half of the book. The rest of the book repeats the material in outlines written by Dr. Craig and several colleagues. The outlines can be used as lecture notes by inservice educators or as guides to study by individuals.

Dr. Craig is professor of medicine and director of the Division of Infectious and Tropical Diseases, University of South Florida College of Medicine, Tampa. He, with David Reifsnyder, M.D., is author of *Departmental Procedures for Infection Control Programs,* also published by Medical Economics Books.

Preface

At one of the meetings of our Tampa-area organization of infection control practitioners, we decided to put together a set of frequently used infection control inservice program outlines to share among ourselves. Since matters relating to infection control always need to be reviewed in hospital-staff continuing-education programs, and since personnel turnover requires that we repeat these programs frequently, this seemed like a useful idea. Accordingly, we drew up a list of 12 commonly presented topics, and volunteers agreed to prepare outlines.

The outlines, which take up the second half of this book, are accompanied by statements of objectives and test questions and answers. Preceding the outlines are more complete, running text discussions, which I prepared for each topic. These chapters, supplemented by reading material listed in the bibliographies, should enable you to communicate good information to your audience and respond knowledgeably to their questions.

The book should help you with the task of providing all your hospital's employees with a fundamental grasp of important aspects of infection control. It is hoped that a subsequent effect might be a decrease in nosocomial infection problems in your institution.

Charles P. Craig, M.D.

1

The role of the infection control practitioner

The original infection control sisters appointed in Great Britain were the predecessors of the infection control nurses—or practitioners—in the United States. Despite the innovating role of British nursing, the specialty has grown and achieved its current status largely in North America. In the early to mid-1960s, the first infection control nurses in the United States were appointed in California. These early nurses functioned principally to gather data about hospital-acquired infections and assist hospitals in developing standards and activities that would meet the requirements of accrediting agencies.

Following the landmark court decision placing hospitals at jeopardy in medical malpractice actions, a flourishing litigation climate fostered infection control as a protective device. Infection control committees, which previously had been relegated to reviewing a few interesting but unusual examples of infections in patients in hospitals, welcomed the presence of infection control nurses who gathered data and information and reported it monthly to the committees. However, the infection control activities were still limited by restricted expectations, a paucity of previous experience on which the practitioners could draw to establish goals for their work, and, in many cases, overlapping assignments for the infection control practitioners, who often also served as nursing supervisors, laboratory technicians, or employee health nurses.

In 1968, the United States Centers for Disease Control began actively urging the nation's hospitals to adopt a more aggressive attitude toward the detection and prevention of hospital-acquired infections. Beginning then, and at an accelerating pace since 1972, the infection control practitioners have become more sophisticated in their activities. Although the improvement is difficult to quantify, many hospitals report a more rational selection of hospital materials based on their effectiveness in infection-generating circumstances, a general decline in incidence of infections in hospitalized patients, improved capability to safely manage increasingly complex illnesses with an acceptable level of infection hazard, and improved employee morale.

These achievements seem to have been generated by a three-pronged attack on hospital infections. The first, the infection control practitioner or nurse, a person with extensive training in microbiology, infectious diseases, environmental sanitation, epidemiology, and administration, is now free to interact with everyone in the hospital, including visitors, administrators, physicians, nurses, engineers, environmental services, and laboratory personnel. The second, the infection control committee, has representatives from medical staff, nursing, and administration and draws upon resource persons from other areas to provide a base of expertise and delegated authority that undergirds the infection control practitioner.

The third, the physician specially trained in the science of hospital epidemiology, is not represented in all hospitals. Where present, the hospital epidemiologist enhances the authority, research, and scientific base of the infection control program.

Areas of responsibility

The modern infection control practitioner has clinical, administrative, and educational responsibilities. In the clinical setting, she or he leaves traditional patient care to the unit nurses, but has daily patient contact while fulfilling her responsibility to be aware of significant patient infections in the hospital. This activity, termed surveillance, includes identification of infections that arise prior to admission to the hospital or are incubating at the time of admission. These community-acquired infections pose significant problems in the hospital because they are frequently caused by microorganisms with significant intrinsic virulence or infectiousness that can spread easily and infect healthy, as well as ill, individuals. They include most of the diseases that require isolation in the hospital: major health hazards such as meningococcal meningitis, tuberculosis, streptococcal infections including scarlet fever and post-streptococcal rheumatic fever, and enteric fevers such as typhoid fever and salmonella food poisoning.

In reality, community-acquired infections are rarely secondarily transmitted within the hospital because there is a high general awareness of their potential for spread. Yet vigilance is required, because on occasion diseases such as hepatitis, salmonella enteritis, and staph wound infections can spread within the hospital or provide reservoirs of organisms that may colonize admitted patients and induce hospital-acquired, or nosocomial, infections.

Nosocomial infections are of greater importance than community-acquired ones because they tend to occur in individuals who have compromised ability to resist infection, are frequently due to organisms resident within the hospital and therefore more resistant to antibiotics, and may be interpreted as signs of careless, indifferent, or scientifically discredited practice by hospital personnel and thus lead to malpractice actions. As a result of analyzing the data she or he collects, the infection control nurse can understand the circumstances within which a particular hospital-acquired infection occurs, the kinds of patients most susceptible to it, and those most likely to spread the infection. She or he may then develop a protocol designed to prevent the spread of the infection. At regular intervals, the data collected by surveillance are collated and analyzed by the infection control practitioner together with the hospital epidemiologist and the infection control committee. Out of such analyses, recommendations for corrective action may then be generated.

Illnesses discovered in hospitalized patients that are of significance for the community at large are reported by the infection control nurse to the local health department. This provides the health department with a readily available sample of the community populace and valid data upon which to establish its community disease prevention and health maintenance activities.

The infection control practitioner is actively involved in employee health programs. Employees may not only be sources of infections for patients, they may acquire infections as a result of their daily contact with infected patients. In smaller hospitals, the infection control practitioner often doubles as the director of the employee health program. In larger hospitals, the practitioner shares responsibility for employee health with a designated health service. Because undetected tuberculosis in employees may be transmitted to patients and other employees, pre-employment chest X-rays and tuberculosis skin testing are of major interest to the infection controller. Other special laboratory testing includes rubella titers for those female employees of child-bearing potential and those who may have contact with infants, children, or pregnant women. Hepatitis-immune status, particularly for hepatitis B, is frequently assessed in individuals who work in especially high-risk areas, such as oncology wards and hemodialysis units. Absence of carrier state for *Salmonella* or *Shigella* may be required for employment of individuals as food handlers in the hospital.

Because of the special knowledge acquired by most infection control practitioners, they can be of value in assessing not only pre-employment health status but the contagiousness of ongoing employee health problems such as viral respiratory infections, infectious rashes, and diarrhea. The practitioner may assist in determining whether an ill employee should have patient contact and help the hospital determine if an employee illness is work-related and therefore compensable under worker's compensation. As local circumstances warrant, special employee health programs may be developed. These may include annual influenza immunization campaigns designed to protect employees and maintain an adequate hospital work force and periodic employee tuberculosis surveillance programs, generally involving tubercular skin testing.

Because immunization standards are rapidly changing, the infection control practitioner should keep the hospital's employee immunization program up-to-date on such complex matters as hepatitis immunization and the TORCH diseases (toxoplasmosis, other diseases acquired in utero, rubella, cytomegalovirus, herpesvirus), so important as causes of congenital illness in infants. Related to immunization is ongoing assessment of employee infection risk in various hospital departments. Examples of high-risk areas include the hemodialysis unit, where hepatitis B is a significant employee risk; the newborn nursery, where congenital rubella may be spread from infants to pregnant nurses; respiratory care units, where undetected tuberculosis in patients may spread to employees; and even the emergency room, where patients with viral respiratory illness can expose and infect ER personnel.

It is apparent that the infection control practitioner has a higher level of awareness of infection hazards in the hospital than any other single individual. Through administrative action, the practitioner translates this awareness into policies and procedures for identifying, monitoring, and, as far as possible, eliminating these hazards. Although the Joint Commission on Accreditation of Hospitals requires infection control policies for every department, some areas of the hospital are clearly more significant than others. In public areas, such as gift shops and snack bars, infection control practices, though not trivial, are not nearly as critical as they are in the intensive care unit, the microbiology laboratory, central supply and receiving, and housekeeping. In these departments, review and construction of infection control policies is an area of high priority for the infection control committee as well as the department directors. The practitioner, because of her or his special education and specific knowledge of the institutional circumstances, is a valuable resource.

A variety of other hospital committees engage in practices related to the infection control program and may use the infection control practitioner as a consultant. Such committees include the audit committee, which frequently selects infectious illnesses for an antibiotic utilization audit; the important policy and procedure committee; the standardization committee, which is charged with reviewing the safety and utility of materials used throughout the hospital; and the head nurses' committee, both a key place to communicate about infection problems and hospital practices and a good listening post from which the infection control practitioner may draw information about emerging problems.

Unless those who need to know find out about them, all the information gathered and policies and procedures developed by the practitioner are of little value. Therefore, educational activities are frequently the heart of an effective infection control program. Education begins with orientation of new employees, so that all will have a basic understanding of the program and of fundamental policies and procedures for isolation in the hospital. As policies and procedures change, infection control update programs must be developed and made available to employees. Reminders are effective educational tools and should be used to reinforce good practice in all areas. The hospital infection control program measures its success by how much the average employee knows about the basic principles of infection control.

The art and science of infection control are dynamic areas that change daily. So the practitioner, too, requires continuing education. In the past few years, several new scientific journals devoted exclusively to infection control have been launched and in each issue include descriptions of new techniques or problem areas. Legislative bodies frequently review and revise their standards concerning hospital infection practices. The effective infection control practitioner spends considerable time in keeping abreast of relevant current literature and government statutes.

A significant portion of this education can be accomplished by attendance at local, regional, and national workshops. Local chapters of the

The infection control practitioner

Association for Practitioners in Infection Control (APIC) schedule regular seminars. State and regional governmental organizations and medical and nursing schools may also sponsor seminars. Nationally, organizations such as APIC, the American Society for Microbiology, the U.S. Centers for Disease Control, and the Infectious Disease Society of America have regular seminars and workshops for infection controllers. Statistics, epidemiology, infectious diseases, medical malpractice, sanitation, and even medical administration are favorite topics. Industry also provides a wealth of teaching activities for practitioners. In many locales, advanced degrees and certification for infection control practitioners are being developed.

Basic principles in infection control

To control the spread of infection it's essential to have a working knowledge of the various types of infectious microorganisms and how they are transmitted. Transmission can be visualized as a chain that begins where infection arises (the source), continues along a route of travel (the vector, or mechanisms of transmission), and ends when it infects a new host (colonization or active infection). Anything that affects the source, vector, or host can contribute to how much transmission actually occurs.

Almost any kind of microorganism can cause hospital-acquired infections. Bacteria are single-celled microorganisms with a hard outer cell wall. They are capable of independent survival outside a host. Viruses, in contrast, cannot survive outside of host cells. They lack the machinery necessary to reproduce. When viruses infect host cells, they take over the machinery of the infected cell and divert it from its normal activities to making new viruses.

Rickettsiae have all the characteristics of bacteria, with one exception: They have lost their ability to survive outside of host cells. Though they have the rigid cell wall of bacteria and a number of independent life and reproductive functions, they cannot totally support themselves or reproduce without some host cell machinery.

Fungi are more organized forms of life than bacteria. Yeasts and molds, familiar to most individuals, are examples of fungi. Although there are hundreds of fungal species, only a few are infectious for humans. Indeed, more fungi provide essential or useful human services than can cause disease. Examples of useful fungi are mushrooms, the yeasts essential for breads and fermenting alcoholic beverages, and the molds that produce many of our antibiotics, including the penicillins and cephalosporins.

Protozoa, like bacteria, are single-celled organisms that can live independently. However, the interior structure of these cells differs in organization and complexity from bacteria; many protozoa do not have a hard outer shell or cell wall and few are important pathogens in humans. Exceptions include the organisms that cause dysentery, malaria, and toxoplasmosis, one of the TORCH diseases.

All infectious organisms exist in reservoirs, or sources from which they may be transmitted to cause infections in new hosts. The most important of these reservoirs are people—including hospital personnel, patients, and visitors. Although water, soil, and equipment may also harbor disease-causing organisms, they are less often the source of infections in hospitals.

In order to get to a new host, the infectious organism must leave its reservoir via a portal of exit. The mechanism whereby this occurs can be easily deduced. If the reservoir is another person, the organisms may be coughed or sneezed out, be shed in stool, urine, or blood, or be shed from the skin during contact between two people or the reservoir person and an instrument.

The vector, or conveyor, of the organism that carries it from the reservoir to the new host is another link in the transmission chain. Certain infections are transmitted directly by immediate contact between two individuals. Some are transmitted indirectly via such intermediaries as a contaminated scalpel blade, scissors, dressings, or even food. Organisms that exist in nature outside of human reservoirs are frequently transmitted to hosts via inanimate objects that we term fomites. Insects may also transmit disease, although this is rare in American hospitals, where insect control is a regular practice. In other parts of the world, yellow fever, malaria, and other insect-borne diseases are transmitted within as well as outside of hospitals. A portal of entry in the new host is the next link in transmission. This is the opening or gate through which the infectious organism gains admission to the host. Certain organisms are introduced only by puncture. These include malaria, yellow fever, and some of the hepatitis viruses. Some may enter through the gastrointestinal tract, such as the virus of hepatitis A and the bacteria of bacillary dysentery. Some, such as influenza virus, enter through the respiratory tract. Broken skin, intravenous lines, Foley catheters, and surgical incisions are other common portals of entry.

The susceptibility of the host is the next link. Individuals have varying degrees of resistance to infection, depending upon whether their natural barriers are intact or are deranged by some illness or procedure. The new susceptible host can be a patient, a hospital employee, or a visitor.

The infection control practitioner

Medications that reduce immunity or the white blood count, surgery that breaks the skin barrier, lung or heart function problems that compromise the lungs' ability to expel organisms—all increase individual susceptibility to acquiring an infection in the hospital. Recognizing susceptible hosts is a major responsibility of all employees, so that special safeguards may be taken.

The final link is the establishment of colonization or infection of the susceptible host. Colonization occurs when a microorganism enters a host and survives and grows there, but does not cause disease. If, as it enters and grows, the organism induces injury in the host, this signifies infection rather than simple colonization.

It should be apparent that the chain of transmission can be interrupted at a variety of points. The most important of these is good hand-washing technique. More diseases are transmitted in the hospital on hands than on any other mechanism. Surprisingly, this extends not only to bacterial infections such as staphylococcal boils and wound infections, but also viral infections such as head colds. The most common mechanism whereby people transmit colds is not by sneezing or coughing, but by touching one another. Most of the organisms transmitted on hands can be effectively removed or neutralized by the use of soap and water.

In certain circumstances, antibiotics can interrupt the chain of infection. Antibiotic therapy of the person who is the source for microorganisms may kill these organisms or render them uninfectious. For example, within 24 hours of beginning penicillin treatment, a person with meningococcal meningitis is no longer infectious for others. Likewise, a strep throat becomes uninfectious 24 to 36 hours after penicillin therapy is begun. Antibiotics may also be given to the susceptible host as a prophylaxis. This is frequently done during surgical procedures that have a high risk of bacterial contamination with a species whose antibiotic sensitivity is predictable.

A variety of isolation precautions may also be used to break the chain of infection transmission. Modern isolation practice attempts to isolate the infection *without* isolating the patient. The goal is to maximize the safety of other patients and personnel while minimizing the interruption of patient care, which can occur under rigid isolation procedures.

Patient placement has recently been formalized so that each patient's status as a source, spreader, or susceptible host of infection is appraised on admission and periodically throughout the hospital stay. Attempts are made to physically separate patients who are major sources and spreaders of infection from those who are most susceptible. Contemporary hospital practice also includes steps to insure that water supply, food, and materials used in patient care are sanitary enough to minimize their role as sources of infection. Patients themselves may participate in infection control if they understand a few basic principles and are adequately educated about their individual status as sources of infection or susceptible hosts. Hospital employees must therefore assume responsibility for keeping their patients apprised of such matters through ongoing efforts at patient education.

Regular examination of patients and chart data by floor personnel is essential so that infection risks may be diagnosed as early as is practical, and steps taken to minimize them. Housekeeping practices are important for infection control. Although bedside stands, windowsills, and floors are not often sources of infection, it should be obvious that if shoddy housekeeping practices are tolerated this situation could change quickly, with major unfortunate consequences. The need for sanitation or sterility in products employed in patient care should be carefully assessed. Items that pierce the body's defenses should always be sterile. Those that pass through body orifices into the respiratory tract or alimentary canal should be sanitized. But those that come into contact solely with intact skin need only be clean.

Goals of infection control program

Involving all hospital people in activities to prevent and reduce the incidence of hospital-acquired infections is essential. On the average, five percent of patients develop nosocomial infections, with rates higher in teaching and federal hospitals and lower in smaller community hospitals. All employees should understand that hospital patients are often compromised in their ability to resist infection while housed in an institution with a concentration of serious infections and are subjected to procedures that ease infection transmission. Invasive procedures, such as starting IVs, break the skin and may deliver contaminated materials directly into the bloodstream. Foley catheters provide a mechanism for retrograde infection of the normally sterile urinary tract. Surgery, because it involves the cutting of skin and mucous membranes, is obviously a major risk factor. Patients may also have underlying metabolic diseases that reduce their ability to resist infection. All of this occurs in a hospital environment replete with infected patients. So it is a testimony to the effectiveness of modern nursing and medical care that the average American hospital has an infection rate as low as five percent or less.

The major goal of infection control programs is to engage all hospital personnel in active infection-prevention measures. Good hand-washing technique before and after each patient contact—and not recontaminating them after washing such as by turning off the faucet with unprotected hands—is the key ingredient in such a program.

Isolation procedures to restrict the spread of community infections, in particular, have been broken down into a number of categories to encourage isolation of the disease but not the patient. Employees should realize that few illnesses require strict isolation. This expensive and patient-isolating practice should be used only when absolutely essential. Protective isolation, in which we attempt to erect barriers around the patient that limit the delivery of infectious materials to him, may seem very useful in concept. But in practice, it has not been found to be of much value to those patients who would most benefit from it. This is probably because individuals such as burn and leukemia patients get most of their infections from bacteria residing in or on their own bodies.

Various wound and skin precautions—called "secretion precautions"—are designed to restrict the spread of organisms from localized and obviously infected surface areas. Enteric precautions are employed to limit the spread of diseases carried in stool and urine. These include bacillary dysentery, *Salmonella* infections, and typhoid. Respiratory isolation is employed for such diseases as influenza and tuberculosis, which can be spread by coughing infectious materials into the air. The principal barrier in respiratory isolation is the mask, which ideally is worn not only by personnel, but by patients. By definition, patients in strict, protective, and respiratory isolation require private rooms in order to accomplish the desired goals. Blood precautions are employed for those diseases largely spread by blood or blood products, most often for hepatitis B.

Another goal of the infection control program is to keep employees aware of the resources available in the hospital to control infection. These include the infection control practitioner and committee, the epidemiologist, the infection control manual, and departmental guidelines. The infection control practitioner provides the link with such outside agencies as the health department and Centers for Disease Control. To supplement educational programs, posted slogans, such as "Wash your hands and drown a germ" and "Nobody ordered an infection—don't deliver any!" can serve as effective reminders.

Bibliography

Association for Practitioners in Infection Control. APIC position paper. *APIC J* 6:9, 1978.

Association for Practitioners in Infection Control Starter Kit. Kenilworth NJ: Schering Corporation, 1978.

Center for Disease Control. *Isolation Techniques for Use in Hospitals* (2nd ed). Washington DC: U.S. Public Health Service, 1975.

Craig CP and Reifsnyder DN, eds. *Infection Control Manual* (4th ed). Tampa: University of South Florida, 1978.

Dunn SA and Johnson M. Education of the new employee: An orientation program for infection control. *APIC J* 5:9, 1977.

2

Gowning, gloving, hand washing, and isolation

Nursing service is the heart of a hospital's infection control program. Although, in the broadest sense, all individuals in a hospital have an important role to play in infection control, the task of the nurses is the most essential. About 60 percent of hospital-acquired infections arise in the urinary or respiratory tract and involve nursing procedures relating to patient position, hydration, urinary drainage, and respiratory care. Most hospital-acquired infections occur as a result of skin-to-skin contact with patients. No other segment of the health-care population has as much immediate contact with patients as nurses, who provide an average of three or more hours of direct care each day to each patient. Through this contact, infectious organisms may be delivered directly to sites where they cause disease, or to sites where they colonize the patient and are subsequently transferred to an infectable area.

It has been observed that those nosocomial infections that are best prevented by careful definition of procedures are also those probably most often transmitted through nursing care. Why this should be so is not clear, but one could speculate that the technical aspects of patient care are not entirely uniform among institutions, being dependent upon design of the facilities, their equipment, staffing patterns, and patient populations. Because these variables may well introduce differences in procedural techniques among the different hospitals, there is a ready opportunity for confusion, nonstandardization, and occasional shortcuts that might expose the patient to increased hazard. Therefore, each institution should carefully consider the peculiarities of its own circumstances in developing policies for nursing care and assure that these policies are communicated to the staff and are followed.

As was stated in Chapter 1, isolation practices are most relevant to community-acquired infections that have great epidemic potential. Since nurses have the widest range of patient contact in the hospital, their training in isolation practices is of paramount priority. Most infections appear to be transmitted through direct person-to-person contact, so hand washing, gowning, and gloving are the key ingredients to restricting infection spread. These important topics are ones with which most hospital personnel have at least a passing acquaintance. For that reason, the educator should seek presentation techniques that will attract an audience and maintain their attention. These topics do not lend themselves so well to a formal lecture presentation as they do to workshops, demonstrations, or the carnival-booth technique in which learning posts to which attendees may circulate are set up in a large room. A measure of the success of an educational program may well be a significant improvement in a hospital's infection-prevention performance.

Gowning and gloving procedures

With a few exceptions, gowning is done to prevent contamination of the clothing or the person of the individual who wears the gown. One exception is the wearing of gowns in the operating room, where a sterile outer covering is necessary to prevent the nonsterile skin or clothing of all personnel from contaminating the wound or instruments. Gowns are also used in protective isolation because they are thought—with little evidence—to prevent transmission of infectious organisms from visitors or personnel to extremely immune-compromised hosts. The same rationale applies to gowns in the obstetric unit or burn unit, where personnel may need to lift and intimately contact patients whose skin has low resistance to infection.

An emphasis on the self-protective role of the gown in most circumstances should be enough to encourage employee compliance; in exceptional circumstances, it may be necessary to carefully enunciate the rationale of gowning. Obviously, in protecting either personnel or patients, the maximally effective gown is long-sleeved, adequate in length, and reasonably resistant to soaking through. The gown worn to protect oneself is likely to become contaminated and therefore should not be worn outside the isolation area lest it contaminate others. Likewise, the gown worn to protect the patient could become contaminated if worn outside the patient care area, and this practice should be discouraged.

Two components of proper gowning that are frequently overlooked are washing hands before gowning and tying the gown securely after donning it. The former practice is sometimes inconvenient because gowns for isolation are kept in the hall outside a patient's room, where there is no readily available hand-washing facility. However, if gowning is done for protection of the patient, as in the nursery or burn unit or protective isolation, it is obviously important that hands be washed prior to gowning in order to restrict contamination of the gown with one's hands. Likewise, if a gown is properly made so that it has long sleeves and a cuff, it is virtually impossible to wash one's hands while gowned without water soaking through the sleeves and cuff, thus negating much of the value of the gown. To avoid hindering patient care, the gown must be fastened on securely. A loosely draped gown will either fall off or inhibit bending over and properly caring for the patient. Like other items of clothing, the gown should not be excessively loose-fitting.

When the gown is removed, it and one's hands should be considered contaminated. If it has been properly worn, the waist-tie can be loosened without contaminating one's clothing. Hands should be washed after this, so that in untying the neck-ties, contaminants are not transferred to the hair or skin around the neck. The gown should then be taken off and turned inside out in the process so that the presumably clean inside becomes the outside when it is folded, rolled, and placed in the proper isolation receptacle. The hands should then be thoroughly washed again to remove any contaminants picked up from the gown while it was being taken off.

Gloving

Except in a few clearly defined areas, gloves, like gowns, are worn to protect the wearer's hands, not the patient. This is important to remember, since the wearer is sufficiently protected with clean disposable gloves which are much less expensive than sterile disposable gloves. Hospital personnel should choose the appropriate glove according to whether gloving is to prevent the hands from contaminating the area being handled (sterile gloves) or prevent soiling of the hands from the materials being handled (clean gloves). It is important to emphasize that gloves are a supplement to, not a replacement for, hand washing. If gloves are worn for any significant period, the bacteria present on the hands will greatly increase and, in the event of a break in the gloves' integrity, pose a real hazard. This hazard is obviously compounded if hands are not washed free of surface bacteria before gloving.

The procedure for gloving, when following gowning and used together with it, is described in the outline. Every attempt should be made to minimize contamination of the exterior of gloves whether or not sterile gloves are used. In the case of nonsterile disposable gloves, only the wrist portion may be touched. With sterile gloves, the skin should contact only the interior of the gloves. If a gown is worn, the glove cuffs should be drawn up over the gown sleeves to provide a more effective protective barrier. If gloves are worn with gown and mask, they are the first to be taken off, then the gown, then the mask. Again, contaminated hands must not touch skin, hair, or clothing.

The mask

In isolation procedures, the mask is worn to prevent personnel or visitors from breathing in particles bearing infectious organisms. One exception to this rule, when the mask is worn to protect the patient, is when personnel or visitors with respiratory infections must have patient contact. Another is when even a few expired respiratory pathogens from an uninfected nurse could spell danger for a patient.

Soiled hands should be washed before touching a mask. On the other hand, if they are already clean, the mask is first put on, then hands are washed before gowning and gloving. The mask is the last item of isolation apparel to be taken off and should be removed only after hand washing. The mask is then to be discarded into an isolation receptacle. There is no justification for wearing a mask from room to room. Masks are cheaper than infections.

Hand washing

Since we know that hands are the most important vector of infectious material in the hospital, hand washing is the single most important method of infection control. A great deal of emphasis has been placed on antibacterial qualities of a variety of hand-washing materials. However, there is no scientific proof that these are superior to simple soap and water. They are licensed for use only because of a theoretical possibility that they might, under certain specific circumstances, be useful. Remember,

16

however, that the qualities that enable certain hand-washing materials to kill bacteria can be toxic for the skin because of these same antibiologic properties. Therefore, it should not be a surprise that individuals who use these scrubs frequently have a high incidence of significant skin reactions, including severe dermatitis and secondary infections of the hands and fingernails. Antibacterial soaps should be restricted to those areas where even low levels of hand contamination pose recognized, or theoretically probable, risks.

If hand washing is to serve its purpose, it is important to avoid recontaminating the hands after washing. This can occur in several ways. An aerator in a faucet may trap organic materials in the water supply, grow various microorganisms such as *Pseudomonas,* and render the water contaminated. If the sink is constructed so that the hands must be held close to the drain where they contact splashed water, or must touch the surfaces of the sink during washing, they can be contaminated after they have been cleaned. If the soap used for hand washing lies in a pool of water, it may very well grow bacteria and be a source of contamination. If towels used to dry the hands are not clean, they can contaminate. If the faucet is grasped with clean, bare, unprotected hands, that obviously contaminated faucet will be a source of recontamination.

In hand washing, there is no substitute for friction. Rubbing two surfaces together in the presence of a good wetting agent and water will very effectively remove surface bacteria. Therefore, good hand-washing technique is to apply adequate friction to all surfaces to remove surface organisms. Since water runs down, one should wash higher areas before lower ones.

Hand washing does not sterilize the skin. The skin contains many peaks and valleys—the pores, hair follicles, and sweat glands. There is no practical way to remove the bacteria that reside in these areas; only surface bacteria can be removed. For that reason, hand washing should be supplemented by the wearing of sterile gloves if sterile tissues or instruments will be handled. The precise procedure for hand washing is well described in the outline.

Isolation practices

While emphasizing the importance of good isolation practices, we should not replace common sense with ritualistic isolation. Good isolation practices combine a careful adherence to procedure and a liberal dose of the common sense that enables one to isolate an infection maximally and a patient minimally.

Gowning, gloving, hand washing, and isolation

Strict isolation

Strict isolation is cumbersome, expensive, and almost always interferes with patient care. There are only 15 entities that require strict isolation. These diseases, such as diphtheria, staph pneumonia, strep pneumonia, and chicken pox, are spread by virtually any route, including direct contact, fomites, air, and intermediate vectors. These are generally community-acquired infections, not hospital-associated, and, therefore, strict isolation needs almost never to be used. Strict isolation for a high fever and an undiagnosed serious illness must be discouraged.

Review of the procedural points in the outline will indicate that strict isolation requires a private room, gowns, gloves, masks, special instruments; special handling of all materials in the room; special management of laboratory specimens; restriction on visiting privileges; extraordinary care in transporting patients, which should be done only under the most urgent of circumstances; and special practices on cleaning of the patient's room after discharge. These alone should be sufficient to discourage unnecessary use of this elaborate level of isolation.

Protective isolation

Despite theoretical considerations that suggest that protective isolation reduces the hazard of infection to patients with uninfected burns, immunosuppressive therapy, lymphomas, leukemia, or severe dermatitis, there are no scientifically valid, carefully controlled studies to document this hypothesis. Indeed, in the case of patients with lymphomas, leukemia, or on immunosuppressive therapy, controlled studies have failed to demonstrate a value for protective isolation. For that reason, many employ a simplified, modified version of protective isolation for such patients, which entails only the wearing of masks and careful hand washing, and perhaps the use of gloves—even these may not significantly benefit the patient. The simplification of procedure saves the time one would otherwise have to take in preparing to care for these patients.

Under exceptional circumstances, such as bone-marrow transplantation or chemotherapy for acute leukemias, the use of a laminar flow or total isolation cubicle for patients, together with carefully selected preventive antibiotics, has been shown to reduce the incidence of infection. However, these are a far cry from the usual protective isolation, and, despite the fact that infections are reduced, patient survival has not been shown to be significantly altered. For these reasons, protective isolation is not commonly used except in burn units and occasionally for patients who have extensive generalized dermatitis.

18

Respiratory isolation

Infection with diseases transmitted by droplets or droplet nuclei, such as tuberculosis, pertussis, and meningococcal meningitis, may be prevented by wearing masks. Because a roommate could hardly be expected to wear a mask 24 hours a day, respiratory isolation cannot be accomplished in a multiple-occupancy room. Since the air of the patient's room may contain a great many infectious organisms, an effective air exhaust system that carries air away from potential susceptible hosts is needed in rooms for respiratory isolation.

These diseases are almost always acquired by breathing in infected droplets or their nuclei, formed when a droplet dries around a contained microorganism such as a tubercle bacillus. It is extremely difficult to acquire the disease from contaminated articles or clothing. Therefore, special precautions are necessary only for inspired air.

Masks owe their protective quality to their baffling effect that traps particles through turbulence and reduces the number inspired to a dose below that necessary for infection. If a mask is torn, moist, or loosely worn, it may not serve this function well.

All diseases requiring respiratory isolation are community-acquired, except under unusual circumstances. Some of them require isolation practices only for a set period, which may be determined by therapy. Measles is infectious for a long time before the appearance of the rash, but only for four days afterward. Meningococcal meningitis is not communicable after 24 hours of effective antibiotics. Whooping cough is no longer communicable after seven days of effective antibiotics. Tuberculosis is not communicable after two weeks of effective therapy. Under unusual circumstances, two patients with the same respiratory disease—proven tuberculosis, for example, may share a room if hospital census demands.

Strict, protective, and respiratory isolation are three categories of infection control that require the isolation of a patient. All other isolation practices are directed to isolating the infection while maximizing the patient's convenience and ability to move about.

Enteric precautions

These precautions are designed to prevent transmission of disease organisms that are excreted in stool or urine and ingested by mouth. Any organism that is excreted in stool and that requires an intermediate host or a period of maturation in soil does not require such isolation. Thus, many parasitic diseases require no specific infection control practices other than normal good hygiene. Other organisms in stool may be too few to induce disease in an exposed individual. Many of the *Salmonella* bacteria, therefore, are difficult to transmit by the direct fecal-oral route; they usually require intermediate residence in foodstuffs, where they may multiply enough to be able to infect other individuals. However, direct transmission may occur in certain high-risk individuals, such as those with sickle-cell anemia or those who have had a gastrectomy. Therefore, enteric precautions are employed in these cases, but no panic should accompany a small break in technique in which a healthy employee experiences a minor exposure.

A recently added indication for enteric precautions is pseudomembranous colitis, a disease that complicates antibiotic therapy. The disease is caused by a species of *Clostridium difficile* which is shed in stool and can survive as a spore in the environment for prolonged periods. It may then colonize other patients and cause disease if they later receive vigorous antibiotic therapy. Because it is frequently difficult to label many forms of hospital-acquired diarrhea, it is probably good practice to use enteric precautions on all hospital diarrheas unless a specific entity, not transmissible by stool, is diagnosed. Patients whose incontinence may lead to heavy contamination of the environment should be placed in private rooms. In all other circumstances, however, a private room is unnecessary.

Certain other diseases are thought, but not proven, to be transmitted by stool. At present, there is debate about the necessity for enteric precautions for certain forms of viral hepatitis, for example, and individual hospital policies should take this into account.

Laboratory specimens from patients on enteric precautions should be appropriately labeled so that the laboratory personnel are not unnecessarily exposed. No special precautions are needed for disposing of simple excreta; local sewage treatment is designed for such a purpose.

Wound and skin precautions

These precautions are necessary for individuals who have extensive wound or skin infections with copious drainage that cannot be adequately contained within dressings. This is one of the isolation categories that may be necessary for hospital-acquired infections, specifically those in surgical wounds. Since infections from such drainage are most commonly transmitted by hands, and occasionally by clothing or fomites, precautions are obviously aimed at restricting these routes. Since the air-borne route is not a problem, masks are unnecessary.

Secretion precautions, a modification of wound and skin precautions, may be used when the infected secretions can be adequately contained within a dressing. The virtue in secretion precautions is that procedures are simpler and the expense to the patient is diminished. In many institutions, secretion precautions may be instituted by members of the nursing staff without a physician order because they neither require patient isolation nor add appreciably to patient expense.

Blood precautions

Blood precautions are used for certain unusual arthropod-borne viral diseases such as the encephalitis caused by viruses carried by mosquitoes, and for viral hepatitis, acquired immune deficiency syndrome, and malaria. Of these, the viral forms of hepatitis are most commonly seen in the hospital. It is important to recognize that hospital employees' risk of acquiring hepatitis other than hepatitis A is related to the site and quantity of their exposure to blood. The risk can be diminished if personnel are forewarned about patients who may be transmitters of hepatitis.

Bibliography

Center for Disease Control. *Isolation Techniques for Use in Hospitals* (2nd ed). Washington DC: U.S. Public Health Service, 1975.

Craig CP and Reifsnyder DN, eds. *Infection Control Manual* (4th ed). Tampa: University of South Florida, 1978.

Dubay EC and Grubb RD. *Infection: Prevention and Control* (2nd ed). St Louis: Mosby, 1978.

Infection Control in the Hospital (4th ed). Chicago: American Hospital Association, 1980.

Mallison GF. The inanimate environment. In *Hospital Infections,* Bennett J and Brachman PS, eds. Boston: Little, Brown, 1979, pp 81-92.

3

Patient placement

In its early form, infection control consisted simply of a list of significant communicable diseases and isolation practices to restrict their spread when infected patients were hospitalized. As hospital infection control evolved, it became apparent that although some isolation practices are probably justified, they had little impact on the incidence of hospital infections. The reason is that the majority of hospital-acquired infections are endemic, rather than epidemic diseases. That is, they are due to the host's own normal flora or opportunists from elsewhere in the hospital environment and occur as single events, not in clusters.

Those infections that derive from the indigenous flora of the host are relatively predictable. But those that arise from the environment vary from institution to institution, and are affected by features such as geographical location, the types of patients hospitalized, local customs of medical management, nursing practice, and institutional antibiotic use. Thus, most hospitals find that the majority of nosocomial infections are due to organisms readily found in the hospital environment, but yet not specifically dealt with in the list of isolatable diseases. In addition, no two hospitals have identical experiences. So a new approach to infection control, embodying a response to particular situations, rather than pre-programmed isolation practices, now seems justified.

One controllable source of infection in the hospital environment that readily comes to mind is other hospitalized patients. A carefully thought-out, situation-oriented intervention program can separate patients with a propensity to spread organisms from patients with a diminished resistance to specific infections. The basic principle of such a patient-placement program is that hospitalized patients can be categorized into three groups: spreaders, high-risk patients with specific resistance defects, and patients not at exceptional risk to either spread or receive infections.

What follows emphasizes the essential elements of any patient-placement program. In practice, it should be adapted to the specific patient population served by a hospital.

Identification on admission

An effective patient-placement program depends upon continuous, prompt, and accurate identification of patients who are potential spreaders of, or highly susceptible to, infection. On admission, patients should be reviewed for specific diagnoses and planned surgical procedures that may give clues to infection risks. For example, a patient who is to undergo prosthetic hip replacement would be recognized as a patient with a high risk of acquiring infection and not placed in proximity to a patient with an active draining infection or pneumonia due to *Staphylococcus aureus* or *Streptococcus pyogens*.

Likewise, a patient whose underlying medical condition is known to decrease resistance to infection should not be placed in a room with a patient who has an active communicable infection. Such at-risk patients are those with leukemia, those undergoing cancer chemotherapy or radiation therapy, those with extensive burns or dermatitis, those with congenital or acquired immune defects in gamma globulin production or function of white blood cells, and those receiving organ transplant.

Coordination and communication

The identification of these patients on admission depends on close communication among various members of the hospital staff. The staff nurse plays a critical role in initial medical evaluation and classification. Nurses should be aware that for many patients admitted to the hospital for specific, predetermined procedures or illnesses, the admitting information fails to describe other unassociated, but important characteristics. For example, an elderly patient may be transferred to the hospital from a nursing home for gallstones, without any written indication on the admission request that he has extensive, draining, staphylococcal decubiti. This information should be obtained in the initial nursing evaluation. Likewise, the nursing evaluation should pick up certain elements of the patient's history that may not be available until the physician's complete history and physical are present in the chart. Key issues, such as a past history of hepatitis or of tuberculosis, should be among those sought in the admission nursing history.

Obviously, if the medical staff of a hospital is aware of the need to promptly communicate infection risks to the nursing staff, the task of patient placement will be simplified. Physicians should recognize that they have a legal responsibility for the outcome when the information they provide for patient placement is incomplete. Malpractice actions have been successfully brought against physicians caring for roommates from whom the plaintiffs acquired infection. Physicians, then, should make every attempt to provide complete information on the health status of patients at admission.

Information about spreaders and at-risk patients within the hospital must be available to the admitting office and bed control personnel. To make logical bed assignments, these people need to know the infection risk or infection status of all patients in the hospital. Nursing personnel in units having a high patient turnover, such as the operating room recovery area, intensive care units, coronary care units, and one-day surgery, should completely assess any patient being considered for transfer so as to assist in proper placement. Controversies, which always arise, should be referred to the nurse epidemiologist whose job it is to study problems associated with patient placement.

The nature of the risk associated with placing different kinds of patients in the same room is not yet well understood for many situations. So what is policy today may very well be eventually discarded based on tomorrow's new information. It's the responsibility of the nurse epidemiologist to keep up with our emerging understanding about how to protect various types of high-risk patients from spreaders.

Classification system

Once relevant information is gathered on individual patients, current classifications can help to identify high-risk patients and spreaders and to place them properly (see Table 3-1). The high-risk susceptible patient has a greater than normal susceptibility to infection. This may be the result of a breakdown of external barriers to microbial invasion, which occurs in burns, dermatitis, wounds, and Foley catheters. Or it may be a deficiency in circulating white blood cells, as in leukemia, or a deficiency in antibodies, as in multiple myeloma or congenital deficiencies. In order to establish a good listing of the hospital's high-risk patients, the practitioner must consider how the body normally resists infection, the routes of transmission of infection, and the minimal inocula of microorganisms necessary to induce infection in normal and compromised hosts.

High-risk susceptible patients should be assigned room space based on an individual consideration of their relative risk to infection, the routes that such infection might take, and the categories of organisms that pose the greatest risk. If no other suitable room is available, these patients should be placed in a private room. Or they may be placed with a medical patient who is neither infected nor likely to become infected, such as a cardiology patient, a surgical patient having clean or clean-contaminated surgery and no active infection, or with other high-risk patients with the same underlying disorder and no infection. High-risk patients should not be placed with a "suspect patient"—one suspected of having an infection or a contagious disease. One special circumstance frequently overlooked is the ease with which an infection in a Foley-catheterized urinary tract can be spread to the collection bag, up the catheter, and into the urinary tract of a roommate who has a Foley in place. Thus, a patient with a Foley should not be placed in the room with another catheterized patient who has a urinary tract infection.

The suspect patient, or the spreader, is a patient who because of infection or incontinence can spread infectious microorganisms actively into the environment. Included in this category are individuals who have draining wounds, active bacterial pulmonary infections, purulent infections of the eye, uncontrolled diarrhea, pneumonia, viral childhood ill-

Table 3-1

Patient placement

	High-risk	Spreader	Clean surgical	Clean contaminated surgical	Contaminated surgical	Infected	Noninfected medical
High-risk	yes	no	yes	yes	no	no	yes
Spreader	no	yes	no	no	yes	yes	yes
Clean surgical	yes	no	yes	if necessary	no	no	yes
Clean contaminated surgical	yes	no	if necessary	yes	no	no	yes
Contaminated surgical	no	yes	no	no	yes	yes	no
Noninfected medical	yes	yes	yes	yes	yes	no	yes

nesses such as chicken pox and measles, or urinary tract infections with a Foley in place. Unless the suspect patient has one of the contagious diseases that require special isolation precautions, he may be placed with any patient who is not at exceptional high risk to infection. Suspect patients should not be placed in the same room with a patient about to undergo clean or clean-contaminated surgery. Patients with recognized contagious disease (confirmed or suspected) or purulent draining wounds, should be placed as specified in the isolation manual listing of disease categories requiring isolation.

Medical patients, for purposes of this categorization, are nonsurgical patients who are not included in any other category. They include patients with such problems as congestive heart failure, acute myocardial infarctions, gastrointestinal bleeding, pulmonary emboli, and kidney stones. If not infected or suspected of being infected, these patients may be housed with a patient in any category who does not have a disease requiring special isolation or precautions.

Classification and placement of surgical patients

Surgical patients should be classified and placed according to the category of surgical procedure they are expected to undergo. Clean surgical patients are those undergoing elective surgery that does not involve an infected or inflamed area, does not open a viscus with large bacterial populations, and is not expected to be drained. They may be placed with any other clean surgical patient, high-risk patient, or noninfected medical patient. Clean surgical patients should not be placed with suspect or infected patients.

Clean-contaminated wounds are those in which the respiratory, alimentary, or genitourinary tract is entered, but there is no unusual contamination. In addition, clean wounds that are mechanically drained are sometimes placed in this category. Such patients may be housed with other patients in this category, with high-risk patients, with noninfected medical patients, or with clean surgical patients, because they do not represent a major risk of spreading infection and are not themselves, unless they have other complicating illness, high-risk patients.

Contaminated surgery patients include those with open, fresh, traumatic wounds and those whose operations are resection of the large bowel with gross spillage, incisions that encounter acute but nonpurulent inflammation, or had a major break in sterile techniques. Examples are cholecystectomy patients with gallbladder cystitis, prostatectomy patients with urinary infection, or appendectomy patients with acute appendicitis.

Patient placement

Such patients may be placed with others undergoing contaminated surgery, or with nonsurgical patients who are not at high risk to infection. However, they should not be placed with clean, clean-contaminated, or dirty surgery, or with patients who have a significant reduction in natural resistance to infection.

Dirty surgery involves old traumatic wounds, those with obvious clinical purulent infection, perforated viscera, or gross fecal contamination prior to the time of surgery. Such patients may be housed with other patients undergoing dirty surgical procedures or with medical patients who are not at high risk of infection.

Not infrequently, exceptions need to be made to the ideal scheme for patient placement. These arise because of inadequate physical facilities, high patient census, the need for specific types of nursing care or special instruments, or even, occasionally, because of patient demand. When an exception is made, it should be understood by all involved that as soon as possible the patient should be transferred to proper accommodations. The reasons underlying the exception should be documented in writing in the chart. Above all, a hospital should not deny necessary medical or surgical care to a patient simply because the ideal scheme of patient placement cannot be satisfied. The final decisions for patient placement should be made by individuals with extensive knowledge in that area, such as infection control nurses, infection committee chairmen, hospital epidemiologists, service chiefs, or hospital chiefs of staff. It is essential to maintain sufficient flexibility in the patient-placement program to accommodate the new ideas and information that appear almost monthly.

Bibliography

Altemeier WA, Burke JF, Pruitt BA Jr, eds. *Manual on Control of Infection in Surgical Patients*. Hagerstown, Md: Harper & Row, 1976.

Cox F. Protective isolation techniques for leukemic patients. *APIC J* 7:21, 1979.

Craig CP and Reifsnyder DN, eds. *Infection Control Manual* (4th ed). Tampa: University of South Florida, 1978.

Golden W. Routine protective isolation: Worth the trouble in neutropenic patients? *JAMA* 242:2045, 1979.

Hyams PJ and Ehrenkrantz NJ. The overuse of single-patient isolation in hospitals. *Am J Epidemiol* 106:325, 1977.

C·H·A·P·T·E·R

4

Urinary tract infection

Five out of every 100 hospitalized patients in this country, according to estimates, acquire a nosocomial infection, and two of these acquire it in the urinary tract. We do not completely understand this high prevalence of urinary tract infection, but we know the importance of such factors as the use of catheters to drain the urinary tract, the prone or supine position, underhydration and decreased urine flow, and incontinence, which, particularly among women, changes the quality and quantity of organisms on the perineum and increases the risk of infection.

In the United States, approximately 400,000 patients a year develop catheter-associated UTIs. Straight in-and-out catheterization to drain urine has an infection rate estimated by most authorities at between one and five percent. Foley catheters have a much higher risk and are responsible for at least half of nosocomial urinary tract infections. If a Foley catheter is open rather than closed at its drainage port, infection of the urinary tract almost invariably occurs within four days. If the system is closed, however, the infection rate in four days is less than 30 percent under circumstances of adequate patient hydration, good sterile placement of the catheter, and good catheter care. At least an additional 25 percent of patients with hospital-acquired urinary tract infections have had other instruments in the urinary tract.

Urinary tract infection

Thus the violation of normally sterile portions of the urinary tract with foreign bodies is the overwhelmingly major cause of hospital-acquired UTI. Such infections are not trivial. They increase hospital stays an estimated five to seven days. Septicemia occurs in one percent of the individuals who develop UTIs, and 30 to 50 percent of this group die as a result. Thus, approximately 50,000 deaths occur each year in the U.S. as a result of nosocomial urinary tract infections.

As many as half of all hospital-acquired UTIs are preventable. Recognizing the risk inherent in putting instruments into the urinary tract and being alert for the signs and symptoms of infection can help prevent disastrous results.

Normal vs. infected urine

Normal urine is a clear amber liquid containing a variety of end-product metabolites and salts. It is excreted by normally functioning adult kidneys in a volume of 1,500 or more ml per day. Cloudiness in freshly voided urine may indicate presence of blood (perhaps from menses contaminating a urine specimen), pus cells, or bacteria. Salts that are normally dissolved, and not visible, in urine may precipitate when an infectious process changes the urine's acidity or alkalinity. Whatever its cause, cloudiness in urine should alert you to a possible infection.

Normally, urine is aromatic but is not excessively unpleasant. When urine has the odor of ammonia it generally indicates severe liver disease with increased circulating blood ammonia, or a breakdown of urea in the urine by bacteria, particularly *Proteus*. Thus, unpleasant odor of ammonia in urine may be a clue to infection.

The microscopic appearance of the urine is important in defining whether an infection is present. Normal individuals excrete up to 300,000 red blood cells each day in the urine. However, since these are divided into 1,500 or more ml per day, in general when urine sediment is examined under the microscope only an occasional red blood cell is seen. If many red blood cells are seen, this may indicate inflammation with disruption of tiny capillaries in the lining epithelium of the urinary tract; a tumor that invades tissues and has abnormal blood vessels that bleed easily; trauma to the kidneys, bladder, or ureters, such as fracture of the pelvis; kidney stones; or glomerulonephritis, an inflammatory disease of the urine-producing structures in the kidney that permits red blood cells to escape into the urine.

Some white blood cells are also normally excreted in urine; one or two white blood cells per microscopic field in urine sediment is not abnormal. However, when more than 10 white cells, or clumps of white cells, are seen in urine sediment, a suppurative infectious process is likely. Such white cells may arise from the tubules of the kidney in pyelonephritis, from the bladder in acute cystitis, or even from the prostate in prostatitis.

Although some bacteria may be excreted in the urine without infection, they are so few that they are not normally seen in a noncentrifuged urine specimen. When the urinary tract is infected, however, there are generally more than 10,000 bacteria per ml of urine, and bacteria can be seen in every highly magnified microscopic field. Thus the observation of bacteria in uncentrifuged or centrifuged urine is strong presumptive evidence for infection. One must keep in mind that a urine specimen improperly collected from a woman may contain bacteria washed from the labia or perineum.

One of the principal functions of the kidney is to conserve water. Under circumstances of large water intake, the kidney excretes water to avoid excessive dilution of the blood. Under fasting circumstances, it retains much water but continues to excrete large amounts of metabolic waste products and salts. Thus, the concentration of urine is high in fasting circumstances and low when there is high water intake. After an overnight fast, urine's specific gravity is usually 1.025 or higher. The concentrating activity of the kidney is rapidly compromised in the presence of kidney infection. Individuals with pyelonephritis generally excrete a urine with a specific gravity of less than 1.015.

Most urinary tract infections arise from the urethra and ascend the urinary tract. Primary development of pyelonephritis from septicemia is unusual but can occur. Because, perhaps, the urethra is short in women and long in men, there is a greater frequency of UTI in women. In general, women have 25 to 100 times as high a risk of UTI as men. Not all UTIs progress and ascend to the kidneys to cause pyelonephritis. As a matter of fact, it is suspected that at least 95 percent of uncomplicated bladder infections in women heal spontaneously without treatment. This is because the bladder itself has several properties that discourage infection, including organic acids in the urine, secretions from the bladder mucosa, and low pH of urine. Also, infecting organisms tend to be washed out when the bladder is emptied. However, if the bladder is vigorously infected, invading bacteria may liberate endotoxins that paralyze the ureters and interfere with their squeezing urine from the kidneys down into the bladder. When this occurs, bacteria can swim up the urine between the kidney and the bladder and infect the kidney to cause pyelonephritis. Certain infections in the kidney may spread to the space around it, causing a perinephric abscess. In the male bladder, urinary infections may spread to involve the prostate (prostatitis).

Urinary tract infection

The urine culture

The *sine qua non* of urinary tract infection is a positive urine culture. To get useful information from a urine culture, the specimen must be carefully collected. This task is relatively simple with a cooperating male, who can simply thoroughly cleanse the glans penis and collect the mid-portion of a stream of urine in a sterile container for culture. With women, the problem is more complex. They collect so-called "clean catch" specimens by holding the labia apart with one hand, carefully washing off the urethral opening on the perineum with soap and water with the other hand, rinsing, still holding the labia apart, and then collecting the mid-portion of a urine stream in a sterile container. However, despite the best technique, up to 20 percent of such specimens become significantly contaminated with organisms from the perineum. Thus, two consecutive urine specimens collected one day apart are necessary to prove infection in a woman.

If collected at the first morning voiding, the specimen contains urine that has been in the bladder overnight. Bacteria greatly increase while in the bladder, so the first morning urine in a person with a UTI generally contains 100,000 or more bacteria per ml. Specimens should be delivered promptly to the bacteriology laboratory in order to prevent overgrowth of organisms. If prompt delivery is not possible, the specimen should be covered with a sterile cap and placed in an ice-water bath where it may remain for no more than one hour until it is delivered.

If the patient suspected of having a UTI has an indwelling Foley catheter, a urine specimen can be drawn from the port designed for this purpose. With the catheter lumen occluded, the flow may be temporarily interrupted and the specimen collected in a sterile syringe. If the patient's Foley catheter has no port, the syringe needle may be inserted in the cleansed flange of the catheter below the sterile water port.

If a patient is incontinent, uncooperative, or otherwise unable to deliver an adequate clean-catch urine specimen, a straight catheter can be used to collect a specimen. The risk of infection is small and acceptable. The mid-stream specimen should be used for culture, with the urine collected in a sterile container and delivered immediately to the lab.

Chapter 7 goes into greater detail with regard to techniques for collecting urine specimens.

Although a voided specimen should contain greater than 100,000 colonies of bacteria per ml to be judged infected, so great a count is not necessary if a catheter specimen is employed. Since the urethra normally contains organisms, even the best voided specimen will generally contain some of them. On the other hand, bladder urine is normally sterile, and therefore even as few as 1,000 bacteria per ml in a catheter specimen is significant.

Symptoms of urinary tract infection

In addition to culture, signs and symptoms are useful in diagnosis of urinary tract infection, and these vary with location of the infection. The acute symptoms of urgency, burning on urination, frequent urination, incontinence, and nocturnal urination with blood in the urine are generally manifestations of infection in the bladder (cystitis). Such patients generally do not have high fever or chills. On the other hand, individuals with isolated infection of the kidneys generally complain of back pain, have high fever (perhaps even the highest of all fevers in adults), chills, abdominal pain, and nausea.

Chronic infection of the urinary tract is entirely different in its symptoms from acute infection. Low back pain, easy fatigability, and, in children, growth disturbances characterize chronic pyelonephritis. Chronic cystitis is associated generally with nocturnal urination, a loss of appetite, and weight loss; it most often occurs in children with anatomic abnormalities of the urethra. Certain individuals have entirely asymptomatic UTIs. This situation is frequently found in pregnant women, many of whom, on careful questioning, reveal they had symptoms earlier but ignored them. It is also not uncommon to find urinary tract infection in patients presenting for a first evaluation for hypertension. The hypertensive kidney seems particularly susceptible to infection.

Causes and prevention of urinary tract infections

Infections of the urinary tract can arise from a variety of sources. In the hospital, poor technique in handling a urinary catheter is often the cause. Hands that are improperly washed and not in sterile gloves can contaminate a catheter and the urinary tract so that active symptomatic infection occurs within the first 24 hours following catheterization. Handling the urine collection bag with hands heavily contaminated with enteric bacteria may contaminate the bag, subsequently the drainage tube and the urine within the bag, and, by retrograde migration, the bladder. Hospital staff should always wash hands carefully before handling a urine collection bag.

It helps to keep in mind that most organisms that infect the urine can swim and may easily enter and move up within a contaminated system, even swimming against the stream in a moving column of water. If a drainage system is left open to the environment, organisms from the air can settle on the end of the drainage tube, multiply there, and migrate up the urine stream into the bladder within two or three days. For that reason, usual practice dictates that opening a closed urinary system should be done only under the most exceptional circumstances, and that all individuals who need continuous urinary drainage should have closed systems.

If irrigations of the urinary tract are necessary to treat bladder stones or following prostate surgery, they are ideally accomplished with a three-lumen catheter rather than by intermittent irrigation, which requires breaking the system. Routine changing of catheters is generally unnecessary and increases the risk of introducing organisms when the new catheter is placed. The most common sign of the need to change a catheter is the presence of calcium deposits in the tubing. These can be easily detected by squeezing the tubing together and rolling it between the fingers. There is a gritty or grainy sensation if calcium deposits are present. Visible salt deposits in the connecting tube also indicate calcium deposits in the catheter. Silicone catheters are slow to accumulate calcium deposits, a considerable advantage if catheterization for more than several days is anticipated.

Since Foley catheters are a major source of urinary infections in hospitals, it's important to avoid their use, except when they are absolutely necessary. They are never to be used solely for nursing convenience. Once it is placed, a catheter should not be manipulated unless circumstances indicate this will reduce complications. Another important preventive measure is to make sure the collection system is never placed so that urine can flow backwards, up toward the bladder. Even under the best of circumstances, contamination of the drainage tubes and bag frequently occur. Since organisms swim more slowly upstream than downstream, urine drainage bags are to be kept below the level of the bladder, but certainly not on the floor where they can become contaminated. Also, since long loops in the urine collection tubing inhibit the free flow of urine, they should be avoided. Valves designed to prevent retrograde flow of urine are not foolproof. It's wise to be skeptical about their value.

A compromised host is at greater risk than the normal host of infection of the urinary tract as well as elsewhere. If an infection does occur, the consequences are also more likely to be serious in the compromised host. If a compromised host must be catheterized, careful attention should be given to adequate hydration to promote good urine flow. The catheterization period must be as short as possible, and the patient ought not to share a room with another catheterized patient who may be infected. Any diabetic who needs Foley catheterization should be considered a compromised patient.

Intermittent self-catheterization, as practiced extensively in many other countries, produces a much smaller risk than Foley catheterization. For many people, it is almost as effective as Foley catheterization in achieving good drainage and preventing incontinence. However, it requires additional nursing care and thus is not practical in all hospital environments. When at home, a trained patient can perform intermittent catheterization himself. Under these circumstances, simple clean technique generally suffices to minimize infection risk. In the hospital, however, where patients are generally sicker and where multiple antibiotic-resistant organisms reside, intermittent catheterization should be a sterile procedure, whether done by personnel or the patient.

Occasionally, leg bags are used for individuals who have neurologic disease that affects bladder function. Although these improve the patient's ability to be ambulatory, they have rather significant drawbacks. The small volume of the leg bags requires frequent emptying, there is no reflux valve, and the bag must be changed each day. For these reasons, breaking the system is very common. Leg bags should be discouraged in hospitalized patients and restricted largely to those at home. If a clean bag cannot be supplied to the home patient every day, a proper cleaning procedure should be developed to prevent the bag from becoming a source of major infection.

In review, urinary tract infections occur with high frequency and account for 40 percent of all hospital-acquired infections. Three-fourths of hospital-acquired UTIs follow instrumentation, principally the Foley catheter. The longer it is left in place, the more likely it is the patient will become infected. If the Foley is left open, the likelihood of infection becomes unacceptably high. Good Foley catheter care significantly reduces the incidence of infection. Minimizing the use of the Foley is the most effective means of reducing the frequency of urinary infections.

Bibliography

Andriole V. Preventing catheter-induced urinary tract infections. *Hosp Prac* 3:61, 1968.

Bard R. Important laboratory values in the practice of urology. *Infec Con Urol Care* 3:3, 1978.

Becker EL. *Kidney and Urinary Tract Infections.* Indianapolis: Lilly, 1971.

Center for Disease Control. Recommendations for prevention and control of catheter-related urinary tract infections. *Nat Nos Infec Stud Q Rep,* nos 1-2:20, 1973.

Urinary tract infection

DeGroot J. Basic principles of infection control and urethral catheterization. *Infec Con Urol Care* 3:5, 1978.

Garner JS. Urinary catheter care. *Nurs 74* 4:54, February 1974.

Kunin CM. *Detection, Prevention, and Management of Urinary Tract Infections* (3rd ed). Philadelphia: Lea & Febiger, 1979.

Sanford JP. Hospital urinary tract infections. *Ann Intern Med* 60:903, 1964.

Stamm WE. Guidelines for prevention of catheter-associated urinary tract infections. *Ann Intern Med* 82:386, 1975.

5

Wound care

The nurse is involved in virtually every aspect of wound care, except that which creates the wound. Whether a wound is traumatic, surgical, or created by thermal energy, assessment, observation, and dressing fall to the nurse. Despite considerable differences in the degree of nursing participation in wound care in different hospitals, it is universally important—for several reasons. First, wound infections themselves have considerable impact on the patient and hospital. They account for at least one-fifth of all hospital-acquired infections. A wound infected patient stays an average of nearly three extra weeks in the hospital, resulting in additional patient expenses that average much more than $10,000 per case. Wound infections also result in debility, disfigurement, and sometimes death of patients, and are a frequent source of medical malpractice litigation.

Nurses are intimately involved in wound care in two basic ways. Frequent observations to correlate the overall health status of the patient with the progress of healing of the wound are the first step. Then there is the requirement to take corrective action when complications arise, such as when a dressing is fouled with excreta or vomit, when there is heavy bleeding into a wound, or when an uncooperative patient manipulates his wound and dressing.

To adequately assess the patient and interpret the observations, it is important to understand the many interweaving factors that determine the outcome of any wound. The impact of the patient's basic underlying

Wound care

health status, the role of the hospital environment, the significance of pre-existing skin trauma (even one so minor as a razor nick), the role of specific topical medications and drains, and the influence of various dressing materials on wound healing are essential elements the nurse must consider. Despite all of this, however, the fact remains that the principal determinant of surgical wound outcome is the skill of the operating surgeon. Although the nurse can make significant contributions to wound healing, no amount of patient education, wound dressing, topical medications, or nutrition can substitute for good surgical technique.

Assessment of the patient

Nursing responsibilities in wound care may be conveniently grouped in four categories: assessment of the patient, selection of dressing material, changing of the surgical dressing, and observation of the wound for complications with action as indicated. Preoperative assessment of the patient should first consider the patient's general health. The roles that extremes of age, diabetes, obesity, immune depression, or active infection elsewhere play in influencing the rate of infection in surgical wounds is well documented. Patients younger than six months or older than 60 years have twice the frequency of surgical wound infections as do those between these two extremes of age when all other factors are equal.

Although the well-controlled diabetic with no complications manages surgery as well as the nondiabetic patient, complications of diabetes are extremely frequent. For example, up to an estimated half of diabetic patients have neurologic urinary bladder dysfunction. Thus the potential for postoperative urinary tract infection is expected to be greater in the average diabetic than in the nondiabetic. Subtle changes in blood supply, particularly small blood vessel patency, may be present, but unrecognized, in the diabetic. So it is important to not only examine the patient for good pulses in all extremities, but also to check such signs as the rate of capillary filling, the presence or absence of hair on the hands or feet, which may be an early sign of diabetic vasculopathy, and the presence of multiple scars on the legs, which indicate frequent unrecognized trauma, an early sign of neuropathy in the diabetic. The dietary and medication requirements of the diabetic patient should be carefully adhered to, avoiding the risks of hyper- or hypoglycemia in the perioperative period. Obesity is another risk factor in both diabetic and nondiabetic patients, and one that is often overlooked. Obese patients have a wound infection rate one and a half to two times that of their leaner counterparts.

Immune depression is of obvious importance. Low-grade contamination of wounds probably occurs in every instance of surgery. The body's immune mechanisms are responsible for neutralizing the relatively few infectious organisms involved in such contamination and preventing infection. If these mechanisms are compromised in any way, the potential for the organisms to increase and cause disease is enhanced.

Active infection anywhere in the body increases the possibility of infection at a surgical wound site. The causes are multiple, including changes in the skin bacterial flora, changes in hydration associated with fever, the role of antibiotics in selecting for resistant organisms, hypoxia if the infection is pneumonia, and infection of the wound through the bloodstream if bacteremia occurs from the remote infected site.

Another major factor to assess in reviewing a patient headed for surgery is the length of the preoperative hospital stay. The risk of surgical wound infection doubles for every three days (beyond the initial three) the patient is in the hospital. The nursing staff can help keep the preoperative stay short. Prompt collection of data needed by the surgeon to plan his procedure is essential. Quick delivery of specimens to the laboratory helps to get prompt results. When a consultant's assistance is requested, he should hear about it right away and know in what room he can find the patient. Medications should be given precisely as ordered, and all procedures ought to be done with appropriate haste so that surgery is not delayed.

Another feature to be assessed in the preoperative period is the timing and nature of skin preparation. It's been demonstrated that preoperative showering with an antibacterial soap diminishes the incidence of wound infections. The technique used to remove hair from the surgical site is very important. If the site is not hairy, no specific preparation should be undertaken. If hair needs to be removed, clipping carries with it the smallest risk of wound infection, use of a depilatory has a slightly higher risk, and a shave prep has by far the highest infection risk. The timing of the skin preparation is also important. If a shave is done more than several hours before surgery, tiny nicks made in the skin may mature to microabscesses. Obviously, making a wound through a site studded with tiny microscopic abscesses is risky business.

Intraoperative risks

A number of intraoperative features may play a role in the incidence of surgical wound infection. The type of procedure and wound is, of course, of greatest importance. Each of the four categories of surgical

Wound care

wounds described by the American College of Surgeons carries with it an expected incidence of wound infection. Clean wounds are those undertaken electively with no obvious infection, inflammation, or trauma, which do not open bacterially colonized viscera, and which are undrained. They have a very low expected incidence of infection, ranging from less than one percent in clean eye surgery to up to five percent in certain complicated procedures, such as prosthetic orthopedics or cardiovascular surgery.

Clean contaminated surgery is that in which organs, such as the birth canal or intestinal tract, are opened without significant gross spillage of contents or wound contamination. They have a somewhat higher expected incidence of infection, ranging from eight to 11 percent. Contaminated surgery, in which obvious contamination of the surgical field occurs from bacteria resident in the surgical site—for example, colon resection—has an expected incidence of postoperative infection of 22 percent or more. Surgery in which gross purulence is present or in which there is massive contamination of the surgical wound from foreign bodies has an extraordinarily high frequency of postoperative infection complication. In many studies it has been found that these dirty wounds become infected about 40 percent of the time.

If a surgical procedure takes more than two hours, the infection risk may be increased by significant drying of wound edges with loss of viable tissues, episodes of hypotension during surgery with diminished blood supply to the wound edges and diminished renal function, and contamination of the wound site from an unrecognized glove puncture—perhaps in more than half of all surgical procedures—or from the air or wound edges. So the length of the procedure is an important factor to assess.

Obviously, if breaks in technique occur, such as tearing a glove, spillage of intestinal contents, or the use of contaminated instruments, the risk of infection is enhanced. Certain complications occurring during surgery can also increase the risk. Foremost among these are massive wound hemorrhage and hypotension with acute renal failure.

If foreign bodies are purposely or accidentally left in the wound, these provide foci for infection. Foreign bodies lack blood supply and therefore are convenient hiding places for infectious organisms, safe from the assault of host defenses and antibiotics. Drains through the surgical incision carry a higher likelihood of postoperative infection than those that are carried through the skin remote from the surgical wound. Open wounds, because of the large exposed area of defenseless tissue, are much more likely to become infected than are closed wounds.

Functions and selection of surgical dressings

Following surgery, trauma, or burns, dressings are frequently placed over wounds. These serve a variety of functions, depending on the circumstances. Dressings are used to protect the wounds from contamination from bedclothes, the air, or even more likely, from the patient's or some other individual's probing hands. Simply covering the wound protects it against such contamination and is particularly important early in wound healing before granulation tissue forms. Dressings are also placed to protect wounds from trauma. If blunt trauma occurs to a wound, tissue devitalization or bleeding may occur, permitting bacteria in the wound to replicate and infect.

Dressings are sometimes also used to provide a controlled degree of pressure on a wound to restrict bleeding. Blood in a wound acts as dead space in which host defense is ineffective and to which antibiotics may not be effectively delivered. Therefore, compression dressing may be used to restrict hemorrhage. Dressings are frequently employed to absorb wound drainage. The drainage may carry out organisms that, if not drained, would grow to cause serious complications. Likewise, wicking drainage away from a wound provides a healthier environment in which the host's tissues may heal.

Some dressings are employed for immobilization. The most obvious of these is the orthopedic cast. Many do not realize that continued motion in an infected or traumatically disrupted area may prevent healing. This has long been known to be the case in infected joints of the body and also in chronic infectious granulomas. Immobilization of such sites facilitates healing of the infection. Some dressings are used for debridement, such as those used for decubitus ulcers and burns. Debridement is necessary because the dead tissues can harbor microorganisms that delay wound healing or cause infection. Dressings are also used to carry medication onto the wound surface. A final use of dressings is to conceal wounds that are psychologically discomforting to patients or other individuals in order to avoid the complications of emotional stress.

In choosing how to dress a wound, the purpose for which it is used is of obvious importance. Dressings come in a variety of forms. Air-occlusive dressings exclude air and moisture from sites where their entry might be disadvantageous. An example is the dressing frequently used over a hyperalimentation catheter. Air-occlusive dressings are convenient for delivering medications to wounds as well. Nonocclusive dressings are much more frequently used. They facilitate the entry of air with its cleansing and nourishing effect on the wound, effectively wick drainage

Wound care

away from the wound, and are useful in debridement. Occasionally, the dressing scheme for a wound may be altered, with an occlusive compression dressing being used immediately postoperatively, and nonocclusive, noncompressing drainage later, after hemorrhage has been controlled and initial granulation has occurred. On the other hand, many wounds have nonocclusive dressings from the outset.

Certain wounds, such as skin grafts and open wounds, are worsened by the use of adhering materials. Adhering dressings might remove the small growing cells of a skin graft or the fibroblasts of a granulating open wound. A nonadhesive dressing is also convenient to change in draining wounds. Achieving the goal of a dry wound depends on how often the dressing can be removed and a clean sterile dressing applied. Certain dressings carry medications. Antibiotic ointments are used occasionally on wounds to prevent bacterial growth. Venous access sites are an example of this application. Digestive enzymes may be incorporated into a dressing in order to liquefy nonviable tissue and facilitate debridement. Topical agents, such as silver sulfadiazine, may be applied to infected burn wounds to assist in control of the local infection.

Tape is used for two reasons: to secure the dressing, and sometimes to exclude air. If tape is to be used only to secure the dressing, it should be used sparingly, so that air may conveniently enter through the dressing, and so that extensive skin injury or patient discomfort does not occur when dressings are changed. If dressings are to be changed frequently, a nonadhesive binder may be preferred to tape.

Aseptic technique in dressing change

When dressings are changed, it is essential to prevent contamination of the wound from instruments or the nurse's hands. Hand washing with care before and after the procedure is critical. No-touch technique should be used for all wounds, clean or infected. Contaminated materials are not to be carried from the periphery into the center of the wound. If soiled dressings need to be removed first, and hands or gloves are contaminated by these, the nurse should wash and reglove before handling sterile dressings.

If the wound has been drained, the drain site is more likely to have bacterial contaminants than the surgical wound and therefore should be changed or dressed after the surgical wound. It is rarely warranted to reinforce wounds that have become saturated with drainage or with patient secretions. Although the reinforced dressing may present a pleasant, aesthetic appearance, the contaminated materials in the underlying dressing provide a focus for growth of organisms that may overwhelm local wound defenses and cause infection or extensive injury to the surrounding skin. Whenever possible, saturated dressings should be removed in their entirety and replaced, using careful aseptic technique.

Observation for complications

Because of the great frequency with which nurses come into contact with individual patients and observe wounds, they have a remarkable opportunity to make valuable observations on patient status. The well-trained nurse examines a patient for early manifestations of infection before the classic signs—redness, pain, swelling, and increased temperature—appear. The cardinal sign of a wound infection is pus, or purulent drainage. When pus is observed in a wound, the nurse is obligated to record that in the medical record and call it to the attention of the patient's physician. Likewise, such observation should always be reported to the hospital's infection control practitioner so that reliable data on infection rates may be gathered. Such data often provide the earliest warnings of large outbreaks or major problems in the operating theater.

Other wound complications, such as bleeding, superficial dehiscence or opening of the wound, or massive opening of the wound with escape of underlying tissues (evisceration), should be promptly reported to the physician and require nursing intervention until he arrives. Any of these observations, any actions taken, and any treatments administered to the patient should be recorded on the patient's chart.

When teaching wound care, it is important to go over the following key points. Every patient should receive a careful assessment prior to, during, and following a surgical procedure. Strict adherence to aseptic technique is essential when handling wounds. The proper selection of dressing materials must be based on an understanding of the need for a dressing in a given patient. Good technique in the care of the wound as well as regular evaluation of the patient for complications following surgery and, if possible, following discharge complete the nursing responsibilities in wound care.

Bibliography

Altemeier WA, Burke JF, Pruitt BA Jr, eds. *Manual on Control of Infection in Surgical Patients.* Hagerstown, Md: Harper & Row, 1976.

Condon RE and Nyhus LM. *Manual of Surgical Therapeutics* (5th ed). Boston: Little, Brown, 1981.

Craig CP and Reifsnyder DN, eds. *Infection Control Manual* (4th ed). Tampa: University of South Florida, 1978.

Cruse PJ and Foord R. A five-year prospective study of 23,649 surgical wounds. *Arch Surg* 107:206, 1973.

Fekety FR Jr and Murphy JF. Factors responsible for the development of infections in hospitalized patients. *Surg Clin North Am* 52:1385, 1972.

Meshelany CM. Post-op wound dressings. *RN* 42:22, May 1979.

Seropian R and Reynolds BM. Wound infections after preoperative depilatory versus razor preparation. *Am J Surg* 121:251, 1971.

C·H·A·P·T·E·R

6

Tracheostomy

The practice of entering the trachea, or the "windpipe" as it is common-ly called, has a long history. Nearly 1,500 years B.C., the procedure was described in the Egyptian papyri. Tracheostomy was held in disrepute for more than 200 years, from the 16th to the 18th centuries, because of the frequency of complications that occurred with the procedure. Its res-urrection followed an enthusiastic report of its effective application in managing diphtheria and, subsequently, preventing respiratory death in patients with poliomyelitis.

Tracheostomy is now used when direct access to the tracheobronchial tree is required to bypass an obstruction at the larynx or higher, to permit removal of copious secretions, and to instill oxygen and medications into the area. Recent innovations and new techniques have improved the ef-fectiveness of tracheostomy, while reducing the incidence of major com-plications. Metal tubes have largely been replaced by newer plastic materials, which seem to be less irritating to the trachea and are easier to use. The plastic tubes are also better adapted to cuffs that, incorporated into the tube and inflated, provide a tighter seal of the trachea, permit-ting more effective mechanical pressure ventilation. Cuffs used with met-al tubes may slide down and partially or completely occlude the tracheostomy lumen, resulting in hypoxia and, conceivably, suffocation.

Tracheostomy tubes come in a variety of sizes, pediatric through adult, and should be selected according to the size of the patient and the indi-cation for tracheostomy. Those that may need to be left in place for a

Tracheostomy

considerable time may have fenestrae (windows) or a flutter valve, which partially closes during exhalation, so that the patient may talk with the tracheostomy in place.

Tracheostomy is a surgical procedure. Except under the most urgent circumstances, it should be performed in the operating room, where adequate lighting, equipment, patient positioning, and sterility can be assured. Bedside tracheostomy can almost always be avoided by temporary use of an orotracheal or nasotracheal tube. After a tracheostomy has been performed, the tube should be tied firmly to the neck to keep it from being coughed out by the patient. This is a particularly disastrous complication when it occurs during the first 24 to 48 hours after the tracheostomy, since the channel through which the tube passes has not matured and may close, suffocating the patient.

The immediate postoperative care of the tracheostomy tube is quite important. A variety of early complications may jeopardize the safety of the patient. Hemorrhage at the site of a recent tracheostomy is not unusual. The blood may run back through the incision into the trachea and cause a violent cough reflex in the patient, spraying blood into the air with every cough. In the patient with recognized hepatitis B, this poses a distinct hazard to people nearby. But in most cases, hemorrhage at the tracheostomy site is more aesthetically disturbing than anything else. Bleeding may often be controlled by removing the gauze dressing around the tracheostomy site and carefully packing a piece of nonadherent gauze into the wound to apply pressure on small bleeding vessels. If this is not successful, the patient has to be returned to the operating room for adequate hemostasis.

Occasionally, air from the incised trachea leaks into the subcutaneous tissues, the mediastinum, or the pleural space. Such episodes are not often of major importance, unless they result in respiratory embarrassment. If the incision of the trachea is accidentally carried too deep, injury to the posterior tracheal wall and esophagus can occur, with formation of a tracheoesophageal fistula. This is an important complication, since it carries with it the risk of aspiration of upper airway and esophageal secretions into the respiratory tract. Damage to nerves controlling phonation may occur during tracheostomy, but this damage is frequently not apparent until the tracheostomy tube has been removed and the patient begins to breathe orally and nasally again. The tube may be positioned too low in the tracheobronchial tree, and indeed sometimes, especially in children, enters one main-stem bronchus, most commonly the right, thus restricting or even preventing ventilation of the left lung. Although such an event is rarely life-threatening, it can cause important complications, such as those related to hypoxia and significant atelectasis of the left lung, and consequent infection.

Early care of the tracheostomy should be directed at detection of these complications and their prevention. Suctioning should not be done as a matter of course, but when secretions are audible or are seen being coughed through the tracheostomy tube. The inner cannula may need to be changed or cleansed at least every two hours early after tracheostomy to keep it from being caked with blood and thick secretions. Adequate humidification, through attached air delivery system or tracheal mask, will prevent formation of dried plugs and epithelium.

The dressing about the tracheostomy site should be changed as often as it becomes visibly soiled with blood or secretions. The site should be treated as any other surgical wound, with careful, meticulous attention to maintaining a clean site with a dry dressing. Every effort should be made to prevent the introduction of foreign bodies, such as lint and pieces of gauze thread, into the site of the tracheostomy. For that reason, special gauze pads cut to fit around a tracheostomy are now available and may be preferable to handmade dressings.

Aspiration past the tube into the lung can be a problem, particularly in a patient who has a nasogastric tube in addition to a tracheostomy tube. In such a circumstance, positioning the patient to minimize the likelihood of aspiration and the use of a cuffed tube may be advantageous. Care should be taken that pressure within the cuff does not extensively damage the epithelium of the trachea. Specific instructions about the volume of air to be introduced to the cuff and the frequency and technique for periodically deflating it should be written in the chart by the attending physician.

A variety of late complications also occur with tracheostomy. Bleeding remains a significant danger. In patients with prolonged tracheostomy, especially metal tracheostomies or cuffed tubes, erosion through the tracheal wall into a major vessel can sometimes result in massive hemorrhage and death. Other complications of injury to the trachea include the formation of fistulas between the trachea and esophagus and the trachea and the skin, stenosis of the trachea by scar tissue, and pain on swallowing associated with post-surgical derangement of tissues in the neck.

A common complication of tracheostomy is infection. Because the tracheostomy bypasses the upper airways with their effective mechanical barriers to organisms, including secretions, cilia, the nasal turbinates, and the epiglottis, microorganisms may be introduced directly into the trachea. Such introduction can occur at the time of surgery, at the time of suctioning if technique is incorrect, by medications introduced into the trachea, by contaminated equipment, or by contamination of inspired air and gases. Aspiration around even a cuffed tracheostomy tube has been shown to occur with high frequency. Thus, bacterial colonization of the trachea occurs almost invariably with tracheostomy. Therefore, careful and continuous attention needs to be given to the tracheostomy site, care of the tube and suctioning, sterility of instilled medications and air, sterility of instruments and equipment, and even proper filtration of expired air to reduce heavy aerosolization into the surrounding environment. A good tracheostomy program will deal thoroughly with each of these requirements.

Infection is distinguished from colonization by four observations:

- the patient has fever unexplained by anything else;
- secretions from the trachea are purulent;
- on gram stain, secretions contain abundant organisms of a uniform appearance; and
- the patient's chest X-ray shows a new infiltrate.

Although any patient may have one or two of these signs, presence of all four in a patient with a tracheostomy can be assumed to indicate pneumonia. On the other hand, a positive culture from the trachea without these signs indicates colonization. When pneumonia occurs, steps should be taken to assure that infection is not spread to other patients.

Despite the best of care, the incidence of infection of the lung in patients with tracheostomy still approaches 20 percent in most studies. Further complicating this depressing figure is the fact that the organisms are frequently hospital-derived and multiresistant. It is not surprising that attendant mortality is considerable.

Care of the tracheostomy

If the patient is conscious, an explanation of what is to be done should always precede tracheostomy care. In the days after the tracheostomy, any manipulation of the apparatus or suctioning evokes strenuous coughing, sometimes accompanied by cough fractures of the rib. Small wonder, then, that the patient becomes apprehensive. Explaining what is to be done and why will frequently allay apprehension and hasten adaptation of the patient to the procedure.

Although suctioning can be accomplished conveniently by one person, changing the cannula sometimes requires an assistant. Particularly in the first 48 hours, it may be useful to have assistance since if the tube should accidentally slip out of the neck, the patient may asphyxiate unless someone helps maintain an adequate airway until the tube can be reinserted. An extra pair of hands can be lifesaving.

Obviously, all equipment necessary for the planned procedure should be assembled before beginning. Careful asepsis is a key to minimizing the frequency and severity of tracheostomy-associated pneumonias. Hands should be washed before caring for a tracheostomy or its attached respirator tubing. From that point on, all materials should be handled with sterile nursing technique.

Any solutions that may be needed, including medications to be instilled and wash and rinsing solutions, should be set up in small, sterile containers. Nothing should ever be put into a bottle of sterile water or medication that might contaminate it. It is far preferable to pour from the bottle into a smaller container, and thus avoid the possibility of contaminating the entire lot. Bottles of cleaning solution, water, and medication should be changed at regular intervals as determined by the infection committee, to avoid their becoming sources of infection.

Sterile gloves are necessary for changing the inner cannula. The cannula should be removed and placed into fresh hydrogen peroxide solution to soak. The tracheal stoma dressing is usually next. If the gloves have been soiled by the cannula, a fresh pair should be donned for this procedure. Sterile sodium chloride solution without preservative may then be instilled into the tracheal stoma to moisten tissue edges. One to 5 cc of sodium chloride are adequate, depending on the size of the patient. This will frequently evoke a cough reflex and may require suctioning. Gloves should now be changed again and cleaning of the inner cannula completed with a brush and pipe cleaners, followed by rinsing in sterile normal saline. The cannula should be inspected carefully to make sure that no lint or particulate matter remains. Then it is reinserted and locked in place.

Obviously, if the patient is on a mechanical ventilator, the procedure needs to be abbreviated and the inner cannula replaced before dressings are changed and the wound irrigated. In no case should the procedure require more than five minutes. If it exceeds that limit, secretions may build up in the lumen of the outer cannula, preventing replacement of the inner cannula.

After the tracheostomy tube has been reassembled, the outer plate should be cleansed carefully with hydrogen peroxide and saline with sterile, lint-free gauze. The skin around the stoma should also be cleansed with either peroxide and saline or an iodophor solution. If ointment has been ordered, it is to be applied around the stoma. If the tracheal tape has become soiled, it should be removed and replaced.

Tracheostomy

Catastrophic accidents can occur during tape replacement if the patient should cough the tube out. Therefore, an assistant may be of value to hold the tube in place while the tape is being replaced. Finally, all dressings should be secured and a notation made in the chart, so there is good documentation of proper care.

During this procedure it is worthwhile to have an obturator at the bedside in case the tracheostomy tube is accidentally coughed out of the trachea. This will be of great value in reintroducing the tube. If disposable tubes are used, the obturator will have been discarded; therefore, a spare tracheostomy tube should be kept at bedside.

Suctioning of the trachea should also be undertaken with careful sterile technique. The nurse explains to the patient what is to be done, washes her hands, and opens the suctioning kit. Sterile gloves should be donned, or a no-touch technique employed. Suctioning should be done over a sterile field, but if this is impractical, at least a clean field is required. The suction tube should be introduced deep into the tracheobronchial tree with the side port open. Then the port is closed and the tube rotated to remove secretions. A suction tube is to be used only once. If more suctioning of the patient is necessary, the tube should be replaced with a clean one.

If secretions are too thick or tenacious to remove, sterile saline free of preservative may be used in small quantities (1 to 5 cc on physician's order) and the patient suctioned again. Following suctioning, the system should be thoroughly rinsed with sterile water from a cup drawn through the system. The catheter is never to be introduced into the sterile water bottle. The cup and its contents should be discarded after each suctioning. The sterile water bottle should not be used for more than 12 to 24 hours. It should then be discarded, even if solution remains.

Medications used for tracheostomy patients should be from unit-dose containers. If multiple-dose containers are used, these should not be moved from patient to patient and should be discarded after 24 hours. Humidification vessels that are open to the air should be changed every 24 hours and resterilized. Those in closed systems, such as disposable humidifier bottles with piped-in gases, may be safely used until empty unless the system is opened or the supply of gases is known to contain even very few microorganisms. In such cases, even disposable, closed nebulizer vessels should be changed every 12 to 24 hours. If a humidification vessel needs refilling, contents of the vessel should be discarded before new solution is added. In most cases, it is also useful to rinse the vessel with sterile water, pour that out, and shake the vessel dry before adding new solution. Meticulous care helps to avoid contaminating the inside of the respiratory support system with bacteria from one's hands during manipulation of these pieces of equipment.

Occasionally, reference is made to routine culturing of patients with tracheostomy. Opinion is divided as to whether this is necessary. If cultures are ordered, techniques described in Chapter 7 should be followed. In all procedures with tracheostomies, steps should be taken to assure that the patient does not contaminate the stoma or apparatus with his hands.

Bibliography

Crow S. Infection control in the critical care unit. In *Proceedings of the Seventh Annual Teaching Institute*. Irvine, Calif: American Association of Critical Care Nurses, 1980, pp. 71–79.

Eickhoff TC. Antibiotics and nosocomial infections. In *Hospital Infections*, Bennett J and Brachman PS, eds. Boston: Little, Brown, 1979, pp 212, 213.

Infection Control in the Hospital (4th ed). Chicago: American Hospital Association, 1980.

Seid AB and Thomas GK. Tracheostomy. In *Otolaryngology*, Paparella MM and Shumrick DA, eds (2nd ed), Meyerhoff WL and Seid AB, ed, 1980, pp 3004–3013.

7

Techniques for obtaining culture specimens

The majority of infections occurring in hospitalized patients are due to culturable microorganisms that can be identified in most hospital laboratories. Among patients admitted to the hospital with fever, 60 to 70 percent are rapidly identified by careful examination and laboratory testing as having bacterial infections. Among the remaining 30 to 40 percent are those who are classified as having fever of undetermined origin. Of these, 35 to 40 percent have culture-demonstrable infections. Bacteria are responsible for more than 90 percent of hospital-acquired infections.

One hardly needs to be reminded of the concern about infection in hospitals. Special committees and staff direct their energies at infection control. Hospital sanitizing and sterilizing activities are directed principally at controlling the bacterial and fungal organisms in the environment. Ten to 20 percent of patients in hospitals harbor infections. Little wonder, then, that cultures are so frequently performed in hospitals. They are of obvious use in determining the cause of a patient's fever. If a patient has disruption of one or more of the normal barriers to infection, it may be useful to obtain cultures to determine whether organisms from the hospi-

Obtaining culture specimens

tal or its personnel have colonized one of his unprotected sites. Cultures may also be used to evaluate the quality of various cleaning or sterilizing techniques. Occasionally, as part of an education program for house-keeping personnel, cultures are performed on surfaces before and after cleaning with an antimicrobial material to demonstrate the effectiveness of the cleaning.

Cultures using spore forms of organisms that are rather resistant to kill-ing are done regularly to check the effectiveness of sterilizers and sterility of certain materials. If a patient receiving an intravenous fluid develops fever, part of that fluid may be cultured to determine if it is contaminated and is then the source of the patient's infection. Formulas made for in-fants in the hospital may be cultured to prove their sterility. Newborns are much more susceptible to infection than adults because their gastro-intestinal tracts lack some of the adult defenses against invasion by bac-teria. Cultures may also be used when an outbreak of infection occurs in the hospital environment. The source may be sought in the inanimate environment (instruments, furnishings, bed linens, wound dressings, and medications) or in the animate environment (hospital personnel, pa-tients, and visitors).

It is important to bear in mind that a culture by itself never proves the presence of an infection. Infection implies invasion of host tissues by or-ganisms, their growth within the tissues, and a response to their growth by the host. Cultures can only demonstrate whether organisms are pres-ent which could be causing infection. But the invasion of the tissue, the growth of the organisms, and the response of the host must be detected by careful examination of the patient. So though culturing can prove the presence or absence and identity of bacteria, it cannot, by definition, tell what role the bacteria are playing in the site from which they were ob-tained. Thus the growth of staphylococci from a surgical wound speci-men, combined with other evidence, such as redness, heat, and purulent drainage, documents a wound infection. If these signs of infection are not present, the culture growth implies only superficial colonization.

Classification of sites to be cultured

The normal status of the site cultured significantly influences the interpre-tation of culture results. If the site is normally sterile (that is, entirely free of microorganisms) presence of bacteria or fungi will be viewed with con-siderably more concern than if they are cultured from a site normally populated with bacteria, such as the throat. Normally sterile, frequently cultured sites include the blood, urine aspirated aseptically from the bladder, spinal fluid, and other internal body fluids, such as pleural, peritoneal, and joint fluids. Bacteria repeatedly cultured from one of these sites provide strong presumptive evidence of an active infection. Similarly, certain materials used in the hospital are assumed to be sterile. These include surgical instruments, intravenous fluid, and medications for parenteral use. If organisms are grown in cultures from these materials, this constitutes strong evidence for contamination.

Sites that normally have bacterial colonization are called normally colonized areas. They are constantly exposed to environmental contamination and support many microorganisms in the normal state without infection. These areas include the skin, the upper respiratory tract, the gastrointestinal tract, and the female lower reproductive tract. Because these areas normally contain many different kinds of microorganisms, it is obvious that *E coli* cultured from the colon, for example, is of much less significance than *E coli* cultured from the blood.

A third category of sites are those that are normally sterile or colonized but, because of temporary circumstances frequently associated with medical care, acquire a bacterial population different from normal but not causing active infection. If one cuts open the skin of an individual and exposes the underlying tissues they will rapidly acquire bacteria on their surfaces. These bacteria come principally from the adjacent skin, but also may come from dressings, from air, or from other materials, such as irrigants or hands that come into contact with the open wound. The isolation of organisms from these sites does not, in itself, constitute evidence of infection, but only of contamination.

Here are some examples of the types of situations in which contamination occurs. After a patient is intubated, the trachea and larger bronchi become colonized relatively quickly. Sequential cultures taken from tracheal secretions within two to three days of intubation begin to yield the organisms normally found in the throat. Under usual circumstances, these contaminating organisms do not constitute proof of infection, but simply unusual colonization. Likewise, after prolonged pressure on one part of the body, circulation may be impaired for a sufficiently long time for tissue to lose viability. The decubitus ulcer that forms is then accessible to microorganisms that digest dead tissue, but frequently do not invade the surrounding viable tissue. In such a decubitus ulcer, contamination is present but infection is not. Another example of contamination may be found in the operating room. It is not unusual to find bacteria in the exposed tissues of surgical wounds. However, numerous studies have shown that the overwhelming majority of such wounds, contaminated during surgery, never become infected.

Obtaining culture specimens

Principles of culturing

Culture technique varies from site to site to maximize the isolation of disease-causing bacteria and minimize collection of colonizers or contaminants. To culture a normally sterile area, elaborate precautions should be taken to avoid introducing microorganisms, which might be colonizing adjacent tissues, into the culture medium. A careful preparation of skin before venipuncture for a blood culture specimen minimizes the chance of collecting skin bacteria in the aspirated blood. Indeed, one technique for assessing the quality of the average blood culture drawn in the hospital is to review all positive blood cultures to determine how frequently skin bacteria, such as *Staphylococcus epidermitis* and diphtheroids, are isolated.

When obtaining cultures from a normally colonized area, remember that the presence of an inflammatory response by the host, including purulence, helps distinguish colonization from infection. So culture areas showing inflammation, where the microorganisms isolated are much more likely to contain those causing the disease than are cultures taken randomly over tissues. Try to obtain the culture from as close to the inflamed tissue as possible. Thus, if a wound is filled with pus, remove the outer portion with a sterile gauze and culture deep within the wound, rather than simply swabbing off the superficial exudate.

This principle also applies to culturing contaminated areas. In a decubitus ulcer, it is important to remove as much of the superficial drainage as possible before culturing and to take specimens close to viable tissues. The reason for this is illustrated by studies of cultures from individuals with chronic osteomyelitis and draining sinus tracts. Cultures taken from the external orifice of the sinus tract frequently contain numerous bacteria. Occasionally none of these is responsible for the bone infection. If a portion of the sinus tract is surgically removed and cultured, fewer species of organisms are isolated, but it is still a mixed growth. If dead bone is removed and cultured, often only two or three species grow, one of which is likely to be the real pathogen. However, if culture is done of living bone taken from an area adjacent to that where bone has died, only a single species is isolated, the one causing the disease.

Of course, in obtaining cultures on the hospital unit it is impractical to remove all dead and necrotic tissue and culture from the advancing margin of infection. But it is certainly practical to attempt to obtain cultures from as close to the site of active infection as possible. So all superficial drainage should be removed before a culture is taken from deep within a draining sinus tract. Likewise, the external canal of the ear should be thoroughly cleaned before culturing purulent drainage from an infected middle ear.

In culturing from areas where contaminating organisms may be present, it is especially important to deliver the specimen to the laboratory as promptly as possible. Many of the contaminating organisms grow more rapidly and luxuriantly in exudate than do the pathogens themselves. If a specimen is permitted to sit for a period before it is cultured, the contaminants may multiply so much that the pathogens are simply overlooked in the laboratory. Many pathogenic organisms do not survive well when dry, so specimens should be kept moist. If an infection has a foul odor to it, it may contain bacteria that do not grow in air or are in fact killed in air. So specimens collected from foul drainage should be protected from the air so that anaerobic cultures may be done.

Finally, it is quite important to protect everyone who will subsequently handle the specimens after collection. Remember that organisms cultured from patients with infections may infect others as well. If a culture is taken from a patient who is isolated, this should be marked clearly on all specimens and requisition slips.

Sputum for culture

The oral cavity normally is colonized with many microorganisms. This is particularly true when a patient has sinus infection or periodontal disease. Therefore, if a sputum specimen is expectorated, a patient should be coached not to expectorate sinus drainage by sniffing it into his throat before spitting. He can help also by cleansing his teeth thoroughly before the collection, if at all possible. Since normal saliva contains organisms, the mouth needs a thorough rinsing before the specimen is collected. The contaminants present in the mouth grow very rapidly at room temperature, so it is imperative that sputum specimens be delivered promptly to the laboratory. Because sputum is collected from the oral cavity, it is best to do several cultures to confirm the presence of a pathogen.

Bronchial and pulmonary secretions increase in volume overnight, so collection of sputum in the early morning hours is more likely to yield an adequate volume—approximately 15 ml—of good pulmonary secretions. Three specimens are necessary to conclusively demonstrate a pathogen.

If a patient is receiving antibiotics, these may be secreted into the sputum and could conceivably interfere with the isolation of pathogenic organisms. The pneumococcus, for example, is very sensitive to many antibiotics frequently used to initially treat patients with respiratory complaints. Thus it is important to note any antibiotics the patient is receiving on the requisition to assist the laboratory in selecting proper culture techniques for optimum results. If an unusual diagnosis is suspected, the laboratory may employ unusual media or culture technology. For that reason, the suspected infection should be noted on the requisition that goes to the laboratory.

A cooperative, conscious patient with a productive cough should always yield an adequate sputum specimen. If a patient can carry out instructions and is producing significant volumes of sputum from the chest, he can be supplied with a toothbrush and dentifrice, a mouthwash, tissues to blow his nose, a sterile sputum cup, and tap water. The patient should brush his teeth, rinse his mouth, gargle with mouthwash, and then finally rinse three times with tap water in order to remove any antibacterial activity of the mouthwash. He can then blow his nose, cough deeply, and expectorate the delivered sputum directly into the sterile sputum cup.

With double-bag precautions and labeled with the patient's isolation status, the specimen can be sent immediately to the microbiology laboratory. The nurse's notes should detail the color, amount, consistency, and odor of the sputum. Documenting a foul odor is particularly important as noted above, since it may indicate a suppurative anaerobic process and perhaps lung abscess.

If the patient has a nonproductive cough, it may be necessary to modify this procedure to induce sputum. This is done by nebulizing normal saline, preferably that used for intravenous administration, rather than injection saline, which may contain antibacterial materials. This procedure to stimulate the patient's cough generally requires a physician's order for a respiratory therapist to nebulize the saline.

Very often a conscious patient with a productive cough will be uncooperative because of confusion or delirium. In this circumstance, the usual collection procedure is impossible. In such a case, it is necessary for the physician to order and assist in collection of a nasotracheal specimen. It is, of course, important to explain the procedure beforehand to the patient or the patient's legal guardian and to document the need. The patient may have to be restrained so he will not interfere with procedures and make the specimen useless.

Gloves must be worn during the procedure. The suction catheter should be attached to a Lukens trap so that the specimen can be collected directly into a sterile container. While the patient is inhaling, the suction catheter is passed through the naris and into the trachea. If this is not done correctly, the catheter may pass into the esophagus or back out into the mouth and become hopelessly contaminated. When the catheter is in place, suctioning is done. If nothing is obtained, the catheter may be disconnected from the Lukens trap and 5 cc of nonpreserved normal saline injected through the catheter into the trachea. This almost always induces vigorous coughing and permits the suction collection of an adequate specimen for culture. Again, the specimen should be adequately and appropriately labeled and packaged and promptly delivered to the microbiology laboratory.

If the patient is unconscious, the same procedure is used as for the uncooperative patient, except that restraints are generally not necessary. If a patient is intubated, secretions can be collected into a Lukens trap through a catheter passed deep into the trachea. If the secretions are too sticky to pass easily through the catheter, a rinse with a small quantity of nonpreserved normal saline may bring a specimen into the trap. In some cases, a physician may attach a syringe to a long, medium-sized intercath and pass this deep into the tracheobronchial tree in order to collect secretions far from the point of intubation and, presumably, closer to the infected site.

Urine for culture

A urine specimen contaminated by microorganisms from the skin is a sure sign of poor technique. Proper technique should always yield a specimen adequate for culture. However, even the best of specimens voided from women patients have organisms that have contaminated the urine as it passed out the urethra and over the associated perineal skin. Therefore, quantitative cultures, in which insignificant contaminants can be overlooked, are most often done on voided urine. This is achieved by sampling urine that has remained in the bladder for several hours. Even if the bacteria from an infected site are few, they multiply rapidly in the urinary bladder. While the urine first excreted into the bladder may contain only 500 to 1,000 organisms per ml, if it remains there for three to four hours, it will contain more than 100,000 per ml. Therefore, the first a.m. urine is generally collected.

There are several exceptions to the rule that more than 100,000 colony-forming units per ml must be present to define an infection. *Staphylococcus* and *Candida* grow slowly in urine, but are recognized pathogens. Therefore, if 10,000 or more colonies of these organisms are isolated from urine, this is presumptive evidence of infection. And if urine collected directly from the bladder through a suprapubic or urethral catheter contains more than 100 colony-forming units per ml, this is strong evidence of urinary tract infection.

59

Obtaining culture specimens

Except when fistulas have formed between the skin or gastrointestinal tract and the urinary bladder, or when Foley catheterization is prolonged, infections of the urinary tract are almost always from single organisms. Therefore, if a culture reveals numerous species of organisms, it probably is evidence of a major contamination of the urinary tract at the time of collection.

In women, the anatomy of the perineum is such that it is quite difficult, if not impossible, to collect a voided urine without some degree of contamination. Because the degree of contamination varies from time to time, and because a single clean-catch urine for culture is only 75–85 percent accurate for women, it is important to do confirmatory clean-catch urine specimens on women with positive cultures. Studies have shown that consecutive voided urines from women may be sterile at one time and contain greater than 100,000 organisms per ml at another, simply because of contamination. Therefore, repeat urine cultures are frequently necessary. One way to circumvent this problem is to collect a specimen for culture by sterile single straight catheterization of the urinary bladder. However, if not performed with care and skill, this technique can lead to infection of the bladder and therefore is reserved for circumstances when a physician orders it.

Hospital procedures for collecting clean-catch urines from women vary, depending upon the materials purchased for that use. In general, these contain a cleaning material for the urethral orifice, cleansing sponges, and a sterile specimen cup. The cooperative patient, properly instructed, can perform the entire procedure herself. The specimen cup should be opened before beginning the procedure in order to avoid interrupting it later on. The woman separates and holds her labia apart with one hand during the entire procedure. With the other hand, she washes the urethral orifice thoroughly with soap and water and rinses well with tap water. She then begins to urinate into the toilet or bedpan and, without stopping the urine stream, introduces the specimen cup into the mid-voiding portion to collect 10 to 15 ml or more of urine. The cup is then moved away from the stream, voiding completed, and the cup closed. The urine cup should be delivered promptly to the lab or placed in an icebath—not a refrigerator—in order to slow the growth of any contaminating organisms from the perineum.

The procedure is similar for a cooperative male patient. The patient opens the specimen cup before beginning the procedure. If he is not circumcised, he retracts the foreskin, because contaminating bacteria are frequently found beneath the foreskin on the glans of the penis. The patient then thoroughly washes the glans with soap and water and rinses it

60

with tap water. He then starts the urine stream and, without stopping it, collects the middle portion in the specimen cup. It should be capped and delivered promptly to the laboratory.

For an uncooperative, unconscious, or bedridden woman patient, a specimen may be collected with a straight catheter if the physician so orders. This procedure always requires strict aseptic technique. The entire set-up should be prepared on a sterile field, and antibacterial soap should be used to cleanse the patient's perineum. An iodophor soap is preferable if the patient has no sensitivity to iodine or seafood. Benzalkonium chloride should be avoided since it may contain *Pseudomonas* contaminants.

Each hospital nursing procedure manual ought to provide instructions on sterile catheterizations. Variations include the no-touch technique, which employs forceps, and the sterile glove technique. In any case, if sponges used in cleaning the perineum are held in a gloved hand, the glove must be considered contaminated. Before the catheter is introduced the gloves must be changed or forceps used. The first and last portion of the urine should be delivered into a sterile basin with the mid-portion—10 to 25 ml—collected in a sterile specimen cup. The specimen must be delivered promptly.

Physician assistance is generally required for a child who is uncooperative. Either straight catheterization or suprapubic aspiration of bladder urine is necessary to collect an adequate specimen for culture.

If a patient has a Foley catheter in place, collection of a specimen is relatively simple. However, it is important that the collector stay with the patient until the procedure is completed. Many times, hospital personnel obstruct the flow of a catheter to collect urine in the bladder for culture, then fail to remove the clamp and return, much later, to find the patient with a grossly distended and perhaps septic bladder.

One way to avoid this complication is to use, instead of a clamp, a rubber band around a kinked connecting tube. Then, if something should interrupt the procedure, pressure in the tube can distend the rubber band enough to permit urine to flow. It is important to remember that the goal is to culture urine from the bladder, not from the tubing. If a specimen of urine present in the tubing is collected, organisms may be cultured which are not from the bladder. Correct procedure is to obstruct the flow high in the tube and draw a specimen from a newly established flow.

Most Foley catheter sets now contain a special port for puncturing with a sterile needle and syringe. If this is not present, a short segment of the rubber tubing should be cleansed with alcohol or iodophor and punctured at an acute angle with the needle and syringe distal to the inflation port. It's important to remember that silastic catheters so punctured will generally leak, and the use of Foley catheter sets with urine collection ports is preferable. The specimen may be delivered to the laboratory in the syringe with needle capped, or it may be delivered into a sterile specimen cup. If it cannot be delivered immediately, it should be placed in an icebath.

Throat culture

In taking cultures from the throat, a normally colonized part of the body, it is important to avoid simply swabbing up and down vigorously over the palate, tongue, tonsils, and back of the pharynx. First, the major areas of inflammation are to be found by careful inspection of the throat with a light. These areas most often show a white exudate and surrounding erythema. These inflamed areas are to be rubbed with the culture swab, with care taken not to touch the tongue. Two swabs should be taken for routine throat culture, one from each tonsil. The swabs are placed in a container and promptly sent to the laboratory.

Wound culture

Unless a wound is new and has recently opened or been incised to permit drainage, it is likely to be heavily contaminated with skin bacteria. Therefore, it's important to carefully cleanse around the wound to remove superficial contaminants before taking a culture. Culture material taken from deep within the wound is more likely to contain pathogens than is that taken from more superficial areas. Wound cultures are done with the no-touch technique—that is, by using instruments to hold dressings and swabs.

The individual taking the culture should wash his hands and put on clean gloves to prevent soiling the hands with bacteria that may be in the dressings. The dressings should be removed and placed in a paper bag for disposal, and not under any circumstance thrown into a wastebasket. After the area around the wound is cleansed with the no-touch technique, the sterile sponges used for this cleansing are placed in the bag with the soiled dressing. After all visible secretions have been removed, a syringe or a swab to aspirate material for culture is placed deep into the wound, with care not to touch more superficial areas. If swabs are used, two samples should be collected, one for anaerobic transport medium and one for aerobic culture. If material is collected in a syringe, after any air in the syringe is expressed, a needle can be attached and capped with a clean rubber stopper. This apparatus can then be transported directly to the laboratory for aerobic and anaerobic culture.

Blood culture

Blood is normally sterile, but surrounding tissues are not. Therefore, to obtain a proper blood culture, it is important to thoroughly cleanse the surrounding tissue to prevent contamination of the needle when it passes through those tissues into the bloodstream. When this technique is used, microorganisms cultured from blood provide rather strong evidence for an infectious disease.

In certain bacteremias, bacteria are constantly present in the blood. In other infections, such as abscesses and pneumonia, bacteria are intermittently shed into the bloodstream, and there is a delay of 30 to 60 minutes between the appearance of bacteria in the blood and the development of fever. Since the peak of bacteremia precedes the peak of fever, the culture should be taken while the patient's temperature is rising, if at all possible.

The materials necessary for blood culture, which should all be assembled before the procedure is begun, include a tourniquet, appropriate blood culture bottles, preferably for both aerobic and anaerobic culture, sterile syringe or vacuum tube, two 22-gauge needles, and skin preparation material, generally iodophor and alcohol swabs.

The tourniquet is applied to the upper arm and a prominent vein located. Using an easily accessible vein minimizes trauma to surrounding skin and the likelihood of contamination of blood. Two iodophor swabs are used to prep the area over the vein. The proper technique is an expanding circular motion. The iodophor should remain in contact with the skin for at least four minutes. If it is necessary to palpate the vein again, it should be done with a finger prepped with iodophor. The aspirating instrument is then introduced into the vein, and 10 cc of blood drawn.

Since the needle used to pierce the skin must now be considered contaminated, it should be replaced with a fresh sterile needle. Five cc of blood from the syringe should be introduced without air into each blood culture bottle, after their tops are prepped with iodophor. The label on one bottle—one for culturing for aerobic bacteria—should bear instructions to introduce air. After the procedure, it is sometimes useful to remove the iodophor from the patient's skin with an alcohol swab to avoid local irritation. The blood culture bottles should be delivered promptly to the laboratory so they may be placed in the incubator.

Occasionally, blood is withdrawn for culture from an indwelling arterial or venous line. In studies of this technique, it has been found that approximately 10 percent of such cultures are contaminated. But when bacteremia is present, such cultures are reliable detectors of infection. If these alternative sites must be used because there is not a good vein for drawing culture, this should be noted on the lab requisition.

Nasopharyngeal swabs

A nasopharynx culture is quite uncomfortable for the patient. The swab must be introduced through the nose and back into the throat. Thorough reassurance of adults will help obtain their cooperation. But if the patient is a child or at all uncooperative, it will be necessary to have an assistant to calm and restrain him.

Obviously, since the nasal passage is not straight, a wooden-handled swab cannot be used for this procedure. A fine wire swab with a dacron head, such as is used for urethral cultures, is appropriate. To limit contamination of the swab with skin organisms around the opening of the naris, a nasal speculum is useful. Both nares should be inspected to avoid using one narrowed by a deviated septum. Then, with the patient supine and breathing deeply through his mouth, the swab is inserted either directly into the nose or through a large nasal speculum until it touches the posterior pharynx. The swab is twisted to obtain pharyngeal secretions on the tip and then withdrawn quickly, but not abruptly. It should be placed in a container and delivered promptly to the lab. Delay may result in overgrowth of nasal contaminants and failure to isolate the pathogens sought in the nasopharynx. This culture is most often used in a search for *Haemophilus influenzae* or *Neisseria meningitidis*.

Nasal cultures

Nasal cultures are not often used to detect disease, but rather to detect the carrier state for organisms that may subsequently cause disease, either in the patient being cultured or in those with whom he comes in contact. Organisms sought by nasal culture include *Staphylococcus aureus, Pseudomonas, Candida,* and sometimes *Aspergillus.* The area swabbed is the skin lining the anterior nares.

It is important to explain the procedure to the patient so that an adequate specimen can be obtained without interference. A dacron-tipped wooden culture stick is the proper specimen collector, one for each naris. The patient should lie supine, and the swab should be inserted only 1 cm, since only the skin area is being cultured. The area should be swabbed in a circular motion, and the swab placed in a container and delivered promptly to the laboratory.

Vaginal cultures

Since, like the throat, the vagina has a heavy normal bacterial flora, isolation of bacteria from vaginal cultures does not in itself constitute proof of disease. Only the isolation of recognized vaginal pathogens in association with classical signs and symptoms of pelvic disease constitutes proof of infection. The major exception to this is the isolation of gonococcus from the vagina, which, although it may not indicate infection, always indicates a carrier state for an important pathogen. The vagina's normal flora are likely to grow quite rapidly in a specimen and obscure pathogens. Therefore, the laboratory should culture vaginal swabs promptly.

It's important to protect the hands from contamination when taking vaginal cultures. Therefore, clean gloves should be worn. There should be good light in order to visualize the area being cultured. With the patient in a lithotomy position, the labia are held apart with one hand and a wooden stick swab with a dacron tip inserted 2 to 3 cm. Swabbing in a circular motion helps collect secretions from the walls of the vagina. The swab is placed in a container and delivered promptly to the lab.

Cervical culture

When culturing the uterine cervix, it is important both to avoid contamination by the vagina and not to culture the mucus plug that may be found within the cervix and contains many vaginal bacteria. With the help of good illumination and a vaginal speculum, the cervical mucus plug should be removed with a sterile swab. Any secretions visible on the speculum should also be removed. Then a third swab should be introduced 1 to 2 cm into the cervical canal, rotated, removed, and placed in a container for culture. If gonococcus is suspected, inoculation of a gonococcus culture plate or bottle should be done at the bedside. Media used for gonococcus culture may be kept warm if the collector keeps the plate or bottle in his pocket while preparing the patient for culture. This will help to preserve the viability of the gonococci, which die rapidly if permitted to cool.

Rectal swab

In culturing the rectum, it's important to bear in mind that the intention is not to culture stool. If a stool culture is necessary, most patients can simply provide a specimen. The perirectal glands, however, frequently contain pathogens, most importantly *Shigella,* and therefore rectal swabs are used. Another indication for rectal swabs is an epidemiologic survey for carrier state for organisms. To obtain cultures promptly from a large group of individuals, one may elect to collect rectal swabs rather than waiting for stool specimens.

A large calcium alginate or dacron swab should be used to collect these cultures. The patient lies on the side with his legs flexed at the hip, or alternatively, bends over a table so that the trunk is at a 90° angle with the legs. A good light is necessary and should be adjusted at this point. Then the person collecting the culture dons gloves and with one hand spreads the buttocks to visualize the anus. The swab should be inserted gently, only 2 to 3 cm in adults and 1 to 2 cm in infants. It's important not to introduce the swab too far and risk perforating the rectal mucosa, particularly in young infants. Swabs should be collected from all four quadrants, with care taken to culture around the entire circumference of the rectum. The swab should then be placed in culture medium and sent to the lab. If stool culture is also necessary, a walnut-sized piece of fresh stool in a sterile container is an adequate specimen.

Eye cultures

Culturing the eye for agents causing conjunctivitis is a valuable procedure. However, many of the medications used topically in the eye contain preservatives that are antibacterial and may obscure important pathogens. Therefore, if at all possible, swabs should be taken before any topical anesthetic or medications have been applied. If the patient has already been treated, it may be necessary for the physician to collect scrapings of the conjunctiva or of the cornea.

In culturing the conjunctiva with a cotton swab, the cornea, which is quite sensitive and relatively easily scratched, should not be touched. The culturer should don gloves that have no talc on them and evert the patient's lower lid with a gloved hand. The everted conjunctiva should be gently swabbed with a calcium alginate or dacron swab, to pick up as much material as possible. To avoid any drying of the specimen, the swab should be delivered immediately to the lab for smear and culture.

Ear cultures

The ear canal is normally populated with microorganisms, among them gram-negative bacteria such as *Pseudomonas,* gram-positive bacteria such as *Staphylococcus,* and many fungi. Therefore swabs from the ear canal are not of great value in diagnosing middle or external ear infection. For middle ear infection, puncture of the eardrum should be performed, and this requires a physician. For cultures of otitis externa, swabs of the canal are frequently used but are subject to great variation in interpretation. Ideally, a specimen is collected by aspiration of lymph fluid, from beneath the skin, but this also requires a physician's skills.

Intravascular line cultures

If a patient who has an intravascular line develops a fever, it is frequently the practice to remove the line, culture it, and start an IV at a new site. This is because many investigators have found that the source of fever in such patients is frequently the IV line itself. However, since the line must be removed through the skin, some bacteria are almost invariably present on the specimen. Therefore, a semiquantitative assessment of bacteria on the line is necessary to determine whether it is infected or has simply been contaminated during removal. For that reason, it is very important to carefully cleanse around the IV site before removing the line.

The individual doing the culturing should wear gloves and have sterile alcohol swabs, sterile scissors, sterile forceps, a suture removal set, blood agar culture plates, and a tube of thioglycollate broth prepared before beginning. All work should be done on a sterile drape. After washing, the individual should don sterile gloves and open the sterile drape. The dressing should be removed and the puncture site carefully cleansed with alcohol swabs to remove, as much as possible, all external secretions. After the alcohol dries, the catheter or needle should be removed and pressure applied over the site to prevent bleeding. The catheter or needle may be placed on the sterile drape.

The inner three inches of a catheter or the needle end may be cut from the remainder of the instrument with sterile scissors and placed on one side of the blood agar plate. With the sterile forceps, this should be rolled once to the other side. Then the cut piece can be placed in a tube of thioglycollate broth. Both plate and broth should then be delivered to the bacteriology laboratory for workup. If the culture discloses more than 15 colonies of an organism on the blood agar plate, this is strong presumptive evidence for an infected IV site. Fewer organisms are generally insignificant.

Culturing nonhuman sources

During a workup of an outbreak, a variety of sources in the hospital may be cultured. Although it is recognized that most hospital-acquired infections come from people and not things, epidemics may spring from contaminated materials, medications, or food. The outline describes the techniques to be employed for culturing those most commonly surveyed, including flat surfaces, tubing, air, IV fluids, and hands (*see* pages 207 to 208). However, whenever environmental cultures are taken, the laboratory director and the epidemiologist should be consulted for specific details about techniques to be employed, and they will very often participate in collection of the specimens to assure that their quality will permit accurate interpretation.

Bibliography

Goldman DA, Maki DG, Rhame FS, et al. Guidelines for infection control in intravenous therapy. *Ann Intern Med* 79:848, 1973.

Lennette EH, Spaulding EH, Truant JP, eds. *Manual of Clinical Microbiology.* Washington DC: American Society for Microbiology, 1974.

Mackowiak PA, Jones SR, Smith JW. Diagnostic value of sinus tract cultures in chronic osteomyelitis. *JAMA* 239:2772, 1978.

Maki DG, Weise CE, Sarafin HW. A semiquantitative culture method for identifying intravenous-catheter-related infection. *N Engl J Med* 296:1305, 1977.

Marchiondo K. The very fine art of collecting culture specimens. *Nurs 79* 9:34, April 1979.

Mikat DM and Mikat KW. *A Clinical Dictionary Guide to Bacteria and Fungi* (3rd ed). Indianapolis: Lilly, 1977.

C·H·A·P·T·E·R

8

Hepatitis

Since the 1967 discovery of the Australia antigen by Blumberg in Aboriginal tribesmen on the Australian continent, there has been an explosion in knowledge about viruses that infect the liver. Hepatitis A, commonly transmitted by contaminated food and water and the most common form of viral hepatitis in the 1940s, has been supplanted by hepatitis B, a viral infection transmitted most often by injection or exposure of mucus membranes to contaminated body fluids. More recently, forms of non-A, non-B viral hepatitis have emerged as important complications of blood transfusion. In addition, nonparenteral transmission of certain of the non-A, non-B hepatitis viruses has been described. Thus, at least four, and very possibly more, distinct viruses with overlapping disease manifestations may constitute the spectrum of viral hepatitis. This chapter provides fundamental information about each of the three known hepatitis viruses and their associated diseases. Table 8-1 contains definitions of terms used in this chapter.

Hepatitis A

The virus of hepatitis A has probably been known longer than any other virus that infects the liver. A disease known as infectious icterus was described by Hippocrates and epidemic hepatitis was widely recognized during the Middle Ages. Under the electron microscope, hepatitis A appears as a tiny, 27 nm sphere-shaped virus close in size to the poliovirus, and smaller than the hepatitis B virus. The virus has been successfully

69

Hepatitis

Useful definitions

Antibody: A protein that is produced in the body in response to entry of a foreign agent. Presence of antibody may result in immunity to the foreign agent.

Antigen: Foreign substance that gains entry to the body and stimulates the production of antibody (for example, hepatitis B virus).

Anti-HAV: Antibody to hepatitis A virus.

Anti-HBc: Antibody to hepatitis B core antigen.

Anti-HBe: Antibody to HBeAg, which may be found in persons with HBsAg or anti-HBs and is not an indicator of immunity to infection. However, presence of anti-HBe seems to indicate that this blood is not highly infectious.

Anti-HBs: Antibody to hepatitis B surface antigen.

Carrier: An apparently healthy individual who is carrying a disease germ that is capable of infecting others.

Chronic active hepatitis: Hepatitis present six or more months with liver exhibiting extensive necrosis.

Chronic persistent hepatitis: Hepatitis present six or more months.

Dane particle: Intact complete hepatitis B virus particle.

DNA polymerase: Enzyme produced during hepatitis B infection. It appears in serum and in carriers correlates with infectivity. Currently, testing to identify this agent is done only in research laboratories.

Fulminant viral hepatitis: A state of hepatitis that is present when liver necrosis causes impairment of synthesis of liver-derived protein and failure to metabolize or detoxify compounds capable of causing encephalopathy.

HA Ag: Hepatitis A antigen.

HAV: Hepatitis A virus.

HBcAg: Hepatitis B core antigen, identified in the core of hepatitis B virus particles.

HBeAg: This antigen has been found only in persons with HBsAg or anti-HBsAg and is an indicator of intact hepatitis B virus particles. It is commonly present in patients with acute hepatitis B, has significance for infectiousness and prognosis in those with chronic hepatitis B.

HBsAg: Hepatitis B surface antigen, the antigen found on the surface of the virus. Formerly known as "Australia antigen" (HAA). HBsAg can be identified in the serum following exposure or during active disease. May persist for variable periods, many years in chronic carrier state. The chronic carrier state may be asymptomatic or associated with active liver disease.

HBV: Hepatitis B virus.

HI B carrier: Person with positive serum HBsAg and no active liver disease and who has had an organ transplant, cancer chemotherapy, or has been on immunosuppressive drugs. This person is potentially a high shedder of virus.

IgM: Immunoglobulin M, which is antibody formed early in a primary infection.

LFT: Liver function tests.

transmitted to chimpanzees and other primates and has recently been grown in virus tissue culture. The abbreviation widely adopted to designate hepatitis A virus is HAV. It is important to recognize that, although hepatitis B virus also infects the liver, hepatitis A and B viruses are entirely unrelated.

HAV may be inactivated in several ways: by heating to boiling for 20 minutes, by 160°C dry heat for 60 minutes, by chlorination, by ultraviolet radiation, and by formalin. The virus is stable at 60°C for one hour, is not inactivated by ether or acid, and is quite stable in cold storage.

Epidemiology

Prior to the 1960s, hepatitis A had a seasonal occurrence, with higher frequency of clinical disease during the fall and winter months. However, since 1966, data collected by the U.S. Public Health Service indicate no seasonal variation. Hepatitis behaves as an epidemic disease after introduction in small, closed situations and occurs in up to 100 percent of exposed susceptible individuals. It may then entirely disappear from the population and not recur until again introduced from outside.

As one might predict, for a disease spread by people contamination, the incidence of hepatitis A is greatest in the developing countries where sanitation is poorest. The disease tends to occur in younger people in whom it often evokes only minor symptoms or none at all. Because of the high frequency of hepatitis A in Latin America and the Far East, travelers to these areas should take special precautions, including prophylactic gamma globulin injections prior to the visit and avoidance of fresh water, ice, and uncooked foods that might harbor human feces-derived hepatitis virus.

In the United States, large serologic surveys have shown that 30 to 40 percent of the population have positive antibody titers to HAV, evidence of previous infection. In adults, the incidence of positive antibody titers is 80 percent. Most of these individuals have no recognized history of the disease. This propensity of HAV to cause subclinical illness is an important attribute for its perpetuation. Another feature of hepatitis A, which contributes to missed diagnosis, is the similarity of the disease to other forms of hepatitis, particularly those due to alcohol, drug, and anesthesia use, and liver disease associated with gallbladder disease. In the presence of these other disorders, it is not uncommon for hepatitis A infection to be overlooked.

Subclinical cases are probably the major source for hepatitis A in any society. Long-term carrier states are very uncommon, and the disease tends to disappear in closed limited populations. Virus shedding proba-bly occurs for up to one month in individuals with asymptomatic infec-tion. This combination of a relatively long period of virus shedding and high frequency of asymptomatic disease is important to the epidemiolo-gy of HAV.

A second significant characteristic of the disease important to epidemi-ology is the increased frequency of asymptomatic cases among young children who acquire hepatitis A. Because the disease has a high fre-quency in institutions where close communal living is practiced, day-care centers and schools for mentally handicapped children tend to be epi-demic multipliers of the disease.

Children acquire the disease because of close contact with other asymptomatically infected children, then transmit the disease to their parents and older individuals in their households who develop symp-tomatic illness. In a recent survey, more than 10 percent of hepatitis A in a large southeastern urban area was traced to disease transmitted into households by children cared for in day-care nurseries.

Mode of transmission

Hepatitis A appears to be transmitted by at least three distinct routes. The most common route is probably from human fecal contamination of food or water. Sources such as water supplies, milk, raw oysters, green vegetables, and other uncooked foods are probably the vectors of trans-mission responsible for the high frequency of hepatitis A in developing countries where the practice of using human feces for fertilizer favors the spread of the virus.

In developed countries, fecal contamination of uncooked foods or those, such as bakery items, handled after cooking may result in spread of the disease. Fecal contamination of oyster beds or of city water sup-plies as a result of improper sewer connections has also caused out-breaks of hepatitis A. In day-care centers, schools, and homes for the mentally retarded, the poor hygienic practices of children, including im-proper hand washing, handling of other children's genitals or soiled clothing, and sharing of food lead to spread of the disease. When these children enter a household, the failure of family members to wash their hands after contact with the children's contaminated clothing or bodies can then spread the disease to the remainder of the family.

Hepatitis A virus enters the bloodstream briefly during the late incuba-tion-early symptomatic periods of the disease. During this time, blood accepted from the individual for transfusion may be a vector for transmission; however, this route is unusual. Urine, on the other hand, frequently contains hepatitis A virus, as does stool, the most common source of infection. The question of whether saliva is an important vector for transmitting hepatitis A is unanswered. Many suspect that the low level of virus sometimes reported in saliva may be introduced from bleeding gums. The highest level of infectious virus in urine, feces, and probably blood is during the incubation period of the disease. After clinical jaundice occurs, less than one-fourth of individuals have infectious virus in their stools. Thus, transmission probably occurs most commonly from asymptomatic individuals still incubating clinical hepatitis A.

Clinical picture

After the hepatitis A virus is introduced into an individual, it enters the gastrointestinal tract where it infects the mucosa of the intestines. The virus then enters the bloodstream and spreads to the liver, where it begins to multiply but not cause symptoms. This incubation period can range from 10 to 50 days prior to the onset of nausea, vomiting, fever, and jaundice. The average incubation period is four weeks, with a range of three to five weeks.

During the incubation period, migratory pain and sometimes swelling in the joints may occur. Later in the incubation period, fever may be prominent with temperatures up to 104°C. Most individuals who develop clinical hepatitis A suffer an early loss of taste for cigarettes and a generalized feeling of malaise. Appetite loss is common, particularly in the one to two weeks prior to the onset of clinical jaundice. Nausea and vomiting occur just prior to, or coincident with, jaundice. Nonspecific abdominal pain and a tender enlarged liver are common.

When the individual develops jaundice, the sclera of the eyes becomes yellow, the urine becomes tea-colored, and the stool develops a clay-colored appearance because bile pigments are not excreted into bile by the infected liver. Also, the infection of liver cells with the virus results in their disruption, and liver enzymes are released into the bloodstream. This is detected by a rise in such enzymes as SGOT, SGPT, and GGTP.

Diagnosis of hepatitis A has recently been simplified by the introduction of specific serologic tests that permit ruling out other forms of hepatitis, particularly hepatitis B. However, without doing specific tests for hepatitis A, it is still possible to confuse hepatitis A with certain forms of non-A, non-B hepatitis.

Hepatitis B is generally excluded by testing blood of the patient for the surface antigen (HBsAg) and antibody to the core antigen (anti-HBc) of

Hepatitis

hepatitis B. One of these two blood elements is almost always present during the acute phase of hepatitis B. However, since antibodies may persist in the blood for years after an infection, antibodies to the core antigen or surface antigen (anti-HBs) do not clearly distinguish between hepatitis A and hepatitis B. If the patient has not been exposed parenterally to blood or blood products during the past six months, infection with hepatitis B is unlikely, although nonparenteral hepatitis B can occur.

When infection with hepatitis A is suspected, it is essential to rule out other diseases of the liver that can cause similar symptoms: infectious mononucleosis, leptospirosis, yellow fever, toxoplasmosis, and, in certain patient populations, cytomegalovirus infection. The specific confirmatory tests that have been recently introduced provide the most solid evidence for active hepatitis A. Individuals with clinical disease almost always have positive antibodies to hepatitis A (anti-HAV) and, during the acute phase, have IgM antibody to HAV. Since the circulating antibody titers rise during the acute disease, acute and convalescent sera showing a four-fold or greater rise in anti-HAV is as useful as measurement of anti-HAV-IgM.

Unlike hepatitis B or non-A, non-B, the course of hepatitis A is typically acute and brief. Moderate to severe illness lasts one to two weeks with nausea, vomiting, fever, and loss of appetite. In an unusual patient the disease may persist for several months, but recovery without any recurrences or long-term effects on liver function is usual. The chronic carrier state occurs in less than 0.5 percent, and mortality from hepatitis A today is also rare.

Isolation precautions

Selecting the proper precaution to use with a patient having hepatitis A depends on your evaluation of the individual's ability and willingness to cooperate with the nursing staff. If the patient is incontinent of feces for any reason, heavy contamination of the environment may occur. Enteric precautions in a private room are probably the best way to manage such an individual. Even if the patient is cooperative and educable and can be taught how to appropriately dispose of stool, enteric precautions are nonetheless needed because of the possibility that other body secretions may be infectious. Gloves should be worn to handle any tubes or instruments that enter the intestinal tract. A double room is permissible, and toilet facilities may be shared if the individual has good personal hygiene and is continent and cooperative. In many circumstances, it may be desirable to have separate toilet facilities.

City sanitation procedures are adequate throughout the United States to render HAV-bearing stool safe, so no special pretreatment of stool is necessary. Since individuals with hepatitis A cease to excrete the virus shortly after they become jaundiced in most cases, the isolation of most patients with hepatitis A may be unnecessary.

Patient teaching

Two points deserve special emphasis with the patient. The first is that the patient's secretions and excretions are potentially contaminated and should be disposed of with care. It is important to stress careful hand washing after using the toilet, maintaining clean toilet facilities, and avoiding toilets shared by many individuals, such as public rest rooms in the hospital. Likewise, teaching the patient the roles of food and water in transmission of the disease should discourage the patient from using public eating facilities and utensils in the hospital.

Prophylaxis

Since up to 80 percent of adults in this country have antibodies to hepatitis A in their blood, most pooled gamma globulin prepared in this country has easily detectable concentrations of anti-HAV. If given prior to exposure or early in the incubation period, this antibody is protective against hepatitis A. Even seven days after exposure, it will significantly alter and diminish the intensity of the clinical course of hepatitis A. Use of this immune serum globulin should be restricted to travelers to undeveloped countries and individuals who have oral exposure to contaminated body secretions or excretions, such as family members and close personal contacts of patients with known hepatitis A. A dosage of 0.03 ml per kg of body weight gives protection for up to three months. The usual dosage administered is 2 cc. Longer prevention, for up to six months, may be achieved by using a larger dose, 5 cc in most adults.

Hepatitis B

The wide-scale occurrence of hepatitis among recipients of a vaccine containing human serum or of plasma from pooled sources during World War II stimulated research into its cause. In 1945, hepatitis was first transferred with ultrafiltered serum, confirming its viral nature. The recognition that the hepatitis that occurred after an injection had a longer incubation period than many cases of noninjection hepatitis led to the distinction between infectious and serum hepatitis. Until 1967, when

75

Hepatitis

Blumberg, in association with other investigators, reported on the Australian antigen, little progress was made. Since then, a rather thorough understanding of the virus, the disease it causes, its spread, and its control has emerged. It is important for the health professional to be familiar with current terminology in hepatitis and to use appropriate abbreviations. Older terminology such as Australia antigen and hepatitis-associated antigen are imprecise and confusing, and should be avoided.

In contrast with the virus of hepatitis A (HAV), which has RNA as its nucleic acid, hepatitis B virus (HBV) is a DNA virus. It is a virus larger than that of hepatitis A and under the electron microscope looks very similar to the herpesvirus. The 45 nm virus has been called the Dane particle, after the investigator who first described it. It contains several component materials. The outer portion of the virus is the so called surface antigen (HBsAg). When HBV grows in cells, it produces more HBsAg than it requires. The excess is liberated by the infected cell as free surface antigen in the form of long thread-like or small circular collections. The virus also contains an enzyme necessary for reproducing its DNA. This enzyme, called DNA polymerase, appears in the bloodstream of infected individuals and also is present with high frequency in those who are chronic carriers of hepatitis B. Another antigen, the so called "e" antigen, is also in the bloodstream of acutely and chronically infected individuals and is associated with intact Dane particles. Another antigen is associated with the DNA of the virus and is called the core antigen (HBcAg). During infection, individuals will develop antibodies to most of these antigens and these can also be measured in the bloodstream.

Hepatitis B virus can be inactivated by heating to 98°C for one minute in serum, by dry heat at 160°C for one hour, by formalin, by glutaraldehyde, by iodine, and by chlorine. The virus remains viable in stored blood for transfusion for prolonged periods. It withstands freezing and is therefore commonly found in whole plasma used to treat hemophilia.

Epidemiology

Because hepatitis B is principally transmitted by blood and blood products, and these are used rather uniformly throughout the year in medical practice, the epidemiology of the disease shows no seasonal variation. In recent years, the Public Health Service has received reports of 50,000 to 60,000 cases of hepatitis B each year. Like hepatitis A, hepatitis B is frequently subclinical. As many as an estimated 90 percent of cases are undiagnosed. Thus, the true incidence of hepatitis B in the United States may be close to 500,000 cases per year.

Certain groups of individuals have a higher frequency of disease than others. There is a clear peak of incidences among individuals between the ages of 15 and 29. There is also a high frequency of hepatitis B among hemophiliacs and individuals who abuse intravenous drugs. There is also a high frequency of hepatitis B in male homosexuals. Although the route of transmission among homosexuals is not clearly established, it seems certainly to be associated with their sexual practices.

Health-care workers have at least twice the risk of community members of contracting the disease. But among health-care workers, incidence varies considerably, depending upon the individual's exposure to blood and blood products (see Table 8-2). There is a high frequency of hepatitis B among hemodialysis technicians, hematology, oncology, and renal unit personnel, dentists, surgeons, individuals who work in intensive care units, and those who work in laboratories where blood or serum are frequently handled.

Serologic surveys among surgeons have indicated that the presence of blood-borne markers for previous hepatitis B increases with age. The incidence exceeds 40 percent by the time surgeons have reached the age of 45. Other physicians having high risk include oral surgeons, pathologists, anesthesiologists, and, of course, nephrologists. A good rule of

Table 8-2_____

Blood products

Deglycerolized red blood cells: Red blood cells to which an approximately equal amount of an 8.6 M glycerol solution has been added. The glycerolized cells are frozen and stored continuously at below −65°C. After thawing, the cells are deglycerolized by the agglomeration technique to prepare them for transfusion.

Fresh-frozen single-donor plasma: Removed from the red cells of whole blood within four hours after collection and stored below −18°C.

Platelet concentrate: Platelets are separated with plasma from red blood cells of whole blood and then concentrated by centrifugation and removal of platelet-poor plasma. These platelets, suspended in approximately 20 ml of plasma, are stored at room temperature until issued for transfusion.

Red blood cells: Packed cells that remain after separation of 200-225 ml of plasma from whole blood.

Whole blood: 405-495 ml of blood collected into either 67.5 ml of ACD-A or 63.5 ml of CPD anticoagulant.

Source: Huggins C. Post transfusion hepatitis and blood components. In *Viral Hepatitis: Etiology, Epidemiology, Pathogenesis, and Prevention,* Vyas GN, ed. Philadelphia: The Franklin Institute Press, 1978.

thumb is to consider that anyone who draws or handles blood or blood products is at risk. In addition, those who work in patient care areas where there is a high frequency of hepatitis, such as hemophilia, hemodialysis, and oncology units, are at increased risk. The highest rates of hepatitis B infection occur among technicians and practical nurses who work in these areas.

In the late 1960s and early 1970s, individuals receiving blood transfusions began to experience an unacceptably high frequency of hepatitis B. This was traced to the common practice of using blood purchased from paid donors in commercial blood banks. This practice has been virtually totally abandoned in the United States, and all donated blood is screened for hepatitis B markers. There has been a subsequent decline in the incidence of hepatitis B. Now only 10 percent or less of the episodes of hepatitis following transfusion are due to hepatitis B. The remainder are mostly due to non-A, non-B viral hepatitis.

Another population with high frequency of hepatitis are recent immigrants to this country from developing nations, especially recent arrivals from Southeast Asia. Large-scale surveys of Cambodian, Vietnamese, and Laotian refugees reveal a high frequency of chronic carrier state for hepatitis B. In Taiwan, hepatitis B is common among pregnant women, and perinatal vertical transmission to infants occurs with high frequency. This results in the chronic carrier state in many of these infected infants and numerous sequelae.

Mode of transmission

There is little or no evidence that hepatitis B is transmitted by contaminated food or water. The virus is present in high concentrations in blood, blood products, semen, urine, tears, saliva, and perspiration. Conclusive evidence of fecal transmission of the disease is lacking and most transmission experiments have failed if the source was feces. Obviously, if blood and blood products taken from individuals with disease or carrier state are frequently contaminated, wound drainage and menstrual secretions are potential sources of infection. These infected materials can transmit the virus to recipients by inoculation, by contact with broken skin, or contact with intact mucus membrane. One case of hepatitis B occurring in a technician followed her splashing contaminated serum into her eye.

Perinatal vertical transmission occurs when mothers have hepatitis B during pregnancy. Infants born of these mothers have a high frequency of carrier state, chronic progressive liver disease, and liver cancer.

The clinical picture

The incubation period for hepatitis B ranges from six weeks to six months. A massive transfusion of hepatitis B virus can result in early clinical signs in several days, but the mean incubation period is approximately 60 days.

During the incubation period, giant urticaria (hives) and arthralgia or arthritis are common. These are not specific for hepatitis B, but can occur in hepatitis A and non-A, non-B hepatitis. The patient complains of rather marked malaise and may have low-grade fever. A loss of taste for cigarettes and appetite for food is common. Vomiting, although it may occur, is not as prominent as with hepatitis A. Most patients report fatigue, and depression is common. Liver enzymes become elevated later in the incubation period. Earlier, hepatitis B antigens and viruses may be detected in blood, but the enzymes are frequently normal. Jaundice has its onset at the conclusion of the incubation period, but disease without jaundice is at least two to three times as common as icteric hepatitis B. The urine is frequently dark and the stool light. The disease runs a variable course, most individuals terminating the acute stage within three to six weeks.

Diagnosis

A variety of specific serologic tests are available for the diagnosis of hepatitis B. Radioimmunoassay tests for surface antigen, core antibody, and antibody to surface antigen are most frequently employed. A new test for "e" antigen has little application during the acute phase of the disease, but is valuable in chronic carriers. The presence of hepatitis B surface antigen in the blood usually indicates that the blood is infectious. On the other hand, anti-HBs simply indicates past infection and a degree of protection against hepatitis B. Immunity induced by injection with anti-HBs is usually not lasting, unless the person is challenged and develops active infection. Most individuals with anti-HBs have no past history of clinical hepatitis. Individuals who work in high-risk areas frequently develop anti-HBs without clinical illness. If sequential measures of anti-HBs are done and a fourfold rise in titer occurs, this indicates recent clinical hepatitis B. A variety of liver enzymes are released from injured cells during hepatitis B. These include SGOT, SGPT, alkaline phosphatase, GGTP, and LDH. None of these are specific for hepatitis B.

Because there is close similarity between the symptoms of hepatitis A and B, the clinical course is not diagnostic of the disease. A history, however, is quite helpful. If the person with hepatitis has been exposed to blood or other contaminated body fluids by the parenteral route or mucous membranes, this strongly suggests hepatitis B. Anyone who has received a blood transfusion or blood products during the last six months is at risk of hepatitis B. Individuals who abuse parenteral drugs, male homosexuals, and health-care workers from high-risk areas are likewise at increased risk, and, if they have symptoms, should be suspected of hepatitis B infection.

The clinical course of hepatitis B is quite variable, but 80 to 90 percent recover completely within three to six weeks of onset of jaundice. The state of an individual's immune system may influence the course of the disease. The disease occurs more severely in individuals with altered cellular immunity. The dose of the inoculum, which is determined by the route of acquisition, may also play a role in severity of disease. One curious observation is that very frequently hemodialysis patients who acquire hepatitis B from contaminated machines have mild or subclinical infections, whereas the technicians who care for them have high frequency of severe clinical illness.

Approximately five to 10 percent of patients become long-term carriers of hepatitis B. The carrier state may last from several weeks to an entire lifetime. Certain types of patients seem to more frequently develop into chronic carriers. These include renal transplant, dialysis, and immune-suppressed patients and neonatally infected infants.

The carrier state may be associated with liver disease. The patient may have chronic persistent hepatitis with mild enzyme elevation but no symptoms and no obvious deterioration of liver function, or chronic progressive hepatitis in which progressive liver destruction occurs. Individuals with chronic persistent hepatitis who have positive HBsAg tests for six months or more frequently have positive anti-HBc, but have low frequency of "e" antigen or DNA polymerase. If an individual has chronic HBsAg, enzyme elevation, "e" antigen, and/or DNA polymerase in the blood, there is high probability of chronic aggressive hepatitis. These individuals also have diminished liver function as evidenced by low serum albumin, a prolonged prothrombin time, and other signs of poor hepatocellular function. Such individuals not only have a worse prognosis, but the presence of "e" antigen or DNA polymerase correlates well with high infectiousness of their blood. For that reason, the commercially available "e" antigen test is frequently used on chronic carriers to determine whether special precautions are necessary in handling their blood and body secretions.

Fulminant viral hepatitis is not necessarily preceded by chronic aggressive hepatitis. About five percent of individuals who develop hepatitis B may develop acute fulminant liver necrosis. Signs of liver failure are predominant. These cases are difficult to manage, treatment regimens are frequently unsuccessful, and about 70 percent of the patients die.

Isolation precautions

Considerable controversy exists around the precautions necessary for hospitalized patients with hepatitis B. More conservative measures include the use of enteric and blood precautions for those who are incontinent, uncooperative, and uneducable, as well as for children. These patients are placed in private rooms and may walk in the hall if they are in clean clothing. They may not use public rest rooms or eating facilities in the hospital. Laboratory specimens from their rooms are labeled hepatitis. Infected children are not permitted to share toys with other children. Because many of these precautions are aimed at preventing contamination with feces, urine, or saliva, many have objected to their rigidity. As was pointed out above, feces are not proven sources of spread of hepatitis B, and urine and saliva are only suspected. For that reason, many advocate only the use of secretion and blood precautions. Others advocate this only for those who show themselves to be cooperative and easily educable.

Under secretion and blood precautions, personnel wear gloves for handling any secretions or excretions, as well as contaminated items and linens. The precautions listed above regarding public rest rooms, eating facilities, toys, and lab specimens apply for secretion precautions as well. Still other infection control people advocate only the use of blood precautions, insisting that blood and blood products are the only important vectors of hepatitis B. All infection controllers agree that blood precautions are necessary for HBsAg carriers. These involve wearing gloves while drawing blood and performing venipuncture, using disposable needles and syringes and disposing of them in an impervious container, and labeling all lab specimens hepatitis.

Patient teaching

Because intimacy appears to be necessary for the person-to-person transmission of hepatitis B, patient teaching is an important mechanism for prevention. Basic concepts concerning communication of the disease via blood, blood products, and probably sexual intercourse should be reviewed. Patients should be taught the necessity of hand washing and should be encouraged not to share items likely to be contaminated with blood, such as towels, razors, toothbrushes, emery boards, earrings, or any other personal care items. Family members should refrain from eating or drinking from common food and beverage containers while patients are in the acute phase of hepatitis B. If the patient needs to prepare food for the family, the patient should taste from a separate dish and utensil in order to avoid possible contamination of the entire batch with saliva. Patients should be taught not to induce bleeding or oozing of body fluids by picking at blemishes or sores, which clearly place others at a greater risk. Women with active or carrier state for hepatitis B should take special care handling menstrual secretion. This includes placing used napkins and tampons in impervious bags so that blood does not contaminate receptacles.

In individuals with active hepatitis or carriers with "e" antigen, special precautions may be used for dishes. Patients may use disposable dishes, but it is perfectly acceptable to use reusables. These should be rinsed with a solution of one part household bleach to 10 parts water and then washed as usual. A dishwasher that reaches 189°F is useful for limiting spread of hepatitis within a family. The home hot water heater may be set to assure adequate temperature. However, this imposes a risk of hot water burns when the water is used for bathing or washing. It is better if the dishwasher has a manufacturer's built-in heater that can boost water temperatures within the unit to 189°F.

For individuals at high risk of spreading the disease (active hepatitis B or "e" antigen positive), separate bathrooms are desirable. If toilet facilities must be shared with others, they may be decontaminated after use by pouring a small volume of bleach into the toilet and washing it with a toilet-bowl brush.

Since hepatitis B may be transmitted during sexual intercourse, and the incidence of the disease is highest among those who have sexual contact with patients, total abstinence is an obvious way to reduce the frequency of transmission. This is frequently unacceptable, so the use of a condom, which reduces the incidence of transmission considerably, is recommended. A third alternative is to give the sexual partner hyperimmune globulin, though proof of the effectiveness of the technique is still incomplete. The concurrent use of hepatitis B immune globulin and a condom provides rather complete protection for a sexual partner.

Because of the high cost of hepatitis B immune globulin (up to $150 per 5 cc), some advocate the use of immune serum globulin (ISG) in which there are considerable quantities of antibodies to hepatitis B. Proof of its effectiveness is incomplete, and some studies have found it totally ineffective. Obviously, many couples in which one partner has hepatitis B continue to engage in normal sexual activities. At the height of the disease this is often not a problem, because patients simply do not feel well enough to engage in sex; however, later on the practice is quite common. Whatever course is determined, it's good to remember that the partner may very well have had significant exposure before clinical illness was discovered, and may have had disease or may be incubating it. At this stage, prophylaxis is of no benefit.

One important piece of information to tell individuals who have hepatitis B is how to handle home items that may be soiled with body secretions. For color-fast fabrics, machine washing in a batch separate from family items is recommended. A one-to-10 solution of household bleach and wash water will inactivate virus, but is not safe for all fabrics. It's therefore important to caution the individual to check the clothes labels to determine whether bleach can be safely used. Hand-washable items should be soaked for 10 minutes in a hot detergent solution with 2 tablespoons of bleach per gallon of water, if the fabric can withstand this treatment. Boiling for 30 minutes effectively inactivates the virus, but many fabrics won't tolerate this kind of treatment.

Hard surfaces contaminated with secretions may be treated with a variety of products. The most convenient is household bleach, but patients should be warned that certain hard surfaces may be discolored by this treatment. Glutaraldehyde is an alternative, but this is somewhat caustic and should be recommended only to patients who are highly intelligent and well motivated to carefully follow instructions. Remember that phenolic and quaternary ammonium compounds (such as Lysol) probably do not inactivate hepatitis B virus.

Personnel safety

Personnel caring for patients with acute or chronic hepatitis B can greatly decrease their risk of infection by certain important preventive measures. The cardinal rules are: Avoid touching puncture wounds with unprotected hands, avoid contacting blood-contaminated materials with unprotected skin, and absolutely avoid mucous membrane contact with blood. Since there is some suggestion that hepatitis B virus may persist in dried blood for short periods, soiling of clothing should also be avoided. Personnel should wear gloves whenever handling blood, blood products, or body secretions. If it is technically possible, they should also wear gloves while doing venipunctures or manipulating intravenous devices. They should wear gowns to protect clothing whenever soiling with blood or secretions may occur.

If an employee has a personal injury or exposure in which blood or secretions suspected of harboring hepatitis virus come into contact with skin or mucous membranes or are on puncturing instruments, the episode should be reported in writing. Such reports may provide the key in determining eligibility for worker's compensation.

If such exposures occur, studies should be done to determine whether the employee is susceptible (free of anti-HBs) and the patient a potential source (HBsAg positive). If a susceptible staff person has contact with a source patient, prophylaxis should be administered.

Two large-scale cooperative national studies have documented that adequate doses of hepatitis B immune globulin (anti-HBs) provides a significant measure of protection against clinical illness. This material is expensive and, therefore, should be administered in only those with proven exposures. One dose should be given within seven days of exposure and a second 30 days later. Although a remarkable reduction in incidence of clinical disease occurs in those so treated, protection is not 100 percent effective. It's important to advise personnel of this fact. In addition, there is some suggestion that some people given anti-HBs simply have a prolonged incubation period followed by clinical illness.

An alternative is to use immune serum globulin, since it does have some antibody to HBV. Some institutions use it for exposures likely to introduce extraordinarily small doses of hepatitis B virus. The dosage and timing are the same as with HBIG. This treatment is of questionable effectiveness and is certainly not as effective as hepatitis B immune globulin. A vaccine for hepatitis B is now available. The vaccine may be restricted to use for high-risk hospital personnel and patients because of cost. It is very effective in inducing protective immunity, as it consists of carefully purified HBsAg.

Safety in work practices is very important. All blood, not just that derived from patients with known hepatitis, should be handled as if contaminated. This includes laboratory standard reagents, which are frequently contaminated with hepatitis B virus. All soiled needles and sharp instruments should be disposed of in a safe manner in containers that are not easily penetrated. Ideally, needles should not be recapped, since most needle injuries appear to occur as a result of carelessness or interruption of personnel while they are putting the cap back on the needle. Used needles should not be broken by hand. If the institution's policy calls for them to be broken, this should be done by a mechanical device. Breaking a needle or the hub off a syringe is likely to send small drops of blood into the air which can then come into contact with mucous membranes. Used IV piggyback needles should be discarded immediately and not taped to an IV pole, where they can transmit disease to an unwary person who grasps the pole and punctures his hand.

Any blood or blood products spilled in the environment should be cleaned up carefully. The person doing the cleaning should wear gloves and should use disposable towels or rags soaked with a virucidal agent such as glutaraldehyde or household bleach. The rag and the gloves should be put into an impervious bag and sent for decontamination or to be destroyed by incineration.

Hepatitis B during pregnancy

Much interest is focused on the problem of the pregnant woman with hepatitis B. There is straightforward evidence that hepatitis B is frequently transmitted to infants. Whether this occurs across the placenta or during delivery, the infant is at high risk of premature birth, chronic disease, liver destruction, and carcinoma of the liver. Previous evidence suggested that hepatitis B was not transmitted during the first or second trimester of pregnancy, but some now believe this is possible, and congenital anomalies may follow hepatitis B early in pregnancy. When the virus is transmitted later in pregnancy, chronic hepatitis frequently ensues in the infant. Later in life, the incidence of liver cancer is increased in such congenitally infected infants.

Newborns may also acquire hepatitis from contaminated amniotic fluid, from menstrual blood of their mothers, from breast milk, or saliva. Therefore, despite negative tests on a newborn infant from a mother with hepatitis B, it is important to use prophylaxis in these children. Most neonatologists administer hepatitis B immune globulin routinely to infants born to mothers with acute or chronic hepatitis B after drawing blood for serologic testing. Obviously, such infants should be managed in the hospital as if they were chronic carriers until results of serologic tests are available. Prompt immunization of at-risk infants with hepatitis B vaccine is advisable.

Non-A, non-B hepatitis

With the development of specific serologic tests for hepatitis A, hepatitis B, leptospirosis, cytomegalovirus, EB virus, and several other miscellaneous causes of hepatitis, it was discovered that a significant portion of individuals with viral syndromes and hepatitis could not be categorized. Initially, it appeared that all of these shared the common feature of a recent transfusion. However, recently, epidemics of viral hepatitis not due to hepatitis A or B have been described, at least one of which was suspected to have been water-borne. These forms of viral hepatitis have been lumped together under the heading of non-A, non-B hepatitis, although there is now sufficient evidence to state with certainty that there are at least two different viruses in this category.

No viral agents have been definitely identified as causing non-A, non-B hepatitis. Tentative identification has been reported, but awaits confirmation. Non-A, non-B hepatitis can clearly recur, thus the strong suspicion that more than one virus is associated with this disease. Since recurrence has followed repeated transfusions, it would appear that there are at least two blood-borne viruses, and probably at least three viruses in the non-A, non-B category.

Epidemiology

The most important of the non-A, non-B infections are those associated with transfusion. Non-A, non-B hepatitis accounts for up to 90 percent of all hepatitis following transfusion; and indeed most cases of non-A, non-B hepatitis occur in individuals with a history of receiving transfusion or blood products.

Mode of transmission

The risk of non-A, non-B hepatitis is perpetuated by the absence of a specific test to determine whether blood contains the viruses. Testing blood units for a liver enzyme (ALT) may reduce the incidence of transmission. Many modes of transmission have been documented for non-A, non-B hepatitis. Most episodes follow transfusions of whole blood, red blood cells, or frozen red blood cells, although episodes have also been reported following transfusion of fresh frozen plasma and platelet concentrate (see Table 8-2). Patients and personnel have developed this hepatitis following needle sticks or puncture wounds from blood-contaminated items, so that this represents a risk to hospital personnel similar to hepatitis B.

There have been outbreaks of non-A, non-B hepatitis transmitted nonpercutaneously. In addition, there is a report of a roommate of a patient with non-A, non-B hepatitis who developed the disease without having had transfusions or puncture wounds.

Clinical picture

The clinical picture on non-A, non-B hepatitis is clouded somewhat by the fact that it probably represents more than one disease. Some individuals refer to short incubation and long incubation non-A, non-B hepatitis. The short is typically that which is nonpercutaneously transmitted, whereas the type that has an incubation period of 30 to 50 days is more often transmitted by inoculation. Again, however, the most important of the syndromes is that which is parenterally transmitted, since it occurs most commonly in hospitalized patients. The clinical course of non-A, non-B hepatitis is similar to hepatitis B, but most often not as severe. A large percentage are anicteric. Of all the forms of viral hepatitis, non-A, non-B progresses to chronic hepatitis most frequently. More than 20 percent, according to some studies, develop chronic manifestations.

Isolation precautions

Since the major route of transmission of hospital-acquired non-A, non-B hepatitis is with blood, precautions must be taken regarding all blood-contaminated material of patients who have this syndrome. There is currently insufficient evidence of nonparenteral transmission to justify other isolation practices. The proper practices for isolation—cleanup of blood spills and handling of excretions and secretions—are listed in the outline and are self-explanatory.

Patient teaching

Patient teaching should emphasize the potential for transmission of this disease by blood that comes into contact with mucous membranes or open wounds. As with hepatitis B, patients should be instructed not to share blood-contaminated or potentially blood-contaminated material. Specifics are listed in the outline. It is important to reassure the family that the risk of acquiring the disease is almost exclusively from entry of contaminated blood.

Prophylaxis and prevention

Prophylaxis is not yet clearly established as a useful practice, though many centers advocate the use of immune serum globulin in doses equal to those used for hepatitis B. When an individual is exposed to non-A, non-B hepatitis, the usual dosage is .06 ml per kilogram of body weight of immune serum globulin, repeated in 30 days.

Prevention is the key to restriction of this disease in the hospital; however, the major preventive technique, identification of contaminated blood units, is not yet possible. In the meantime, care should be taken in handling all blood, treating it as if it were contaminated. All personnel should be alerted to any patient with a history of drug abuse or receipt of blood products in the last six months and should observe such a patient for possible disease. In caring for patients who have non-A, non-B hepatitis, staff should protect themselves and others from contact with blood or blood-contaminated body secretions.

Bibliography

Aach RD. Viral hepatitis—A to e. *Med Clin North Am* 62:59, 1978.

Bates HM. Measurement of antibody to hepatitis A virus by RIA. *Lab Man* 16:43, July 1978.

Bond WW, Petersen NJ, Favero MS. Viral hepatitis B: Aspects of environmental control. *Health Lab Sci* 14:235, 1977.

Center for Disease Control. *Hepatitis Surveillance.* Atlanta: U.S. Public Health Service, quarterly reports.

Center for Disease Control. Prospectives on the control of viral hepatitis, type B. *MMWR* Supplement, May 1976.

Center for Disease Control. *Viral Hepatitis: Investigation and Control.* Atlanta: U.S. Public Health Service, Nov 1977.

Feinman SV, Berris B, Sinclair JC, et al. Practical guidelines for assessing patients positive for hepatitis B surface antigen. *Can Med Assoc J* 115:991, 1976.

Gerety RJ and Schweitzer IL. Viral hepatitis type B during pregnancy, the neonatal period, and infancy. *J Pediatr* 90:368, 1977.

Levy BS, Harris JC, Smith JL, et al. Hepatitis B in ward and clinical laboratory employees of a general hospital. *Am J Epidemiol* 106:330, 1977.

Maynard JE. Hepatitis A. *Yale J Biol Med* 49:227, 1976.

Melnick JL, Dreesman GR, Hollinger FB. Approaching the control of viral hepatitis type B. *J Infect Dis* 133:210, 1976.

Naulty JS, Reves JG, Tobey RE, et al. Hepatitis and operating-room personnel: An approach to diagnosis and management. *Anesth Analg* 56:366, 1977.

Prince AM, Szmuness W, Mann MK, et al. Hepatitis B immune globulin: Final report of a controlled, multicenter trial of efficacy in prevention of dialysis-associated hepatitis. *J Infect Dis* 137:131, 1978.

Purcell RH. The viral hepatitides. *Hosp Prac* 13:51, 1978.

Rakela J and Mosley JW. Fecal excretion of hepatitis A virus in humans. *J Infect Dis* 135:933, 1977.

Redeker AG, Mosley JW, Gocke DJ, et al. Hepatitis B immune globulin as a prophylactic measure for spouses exposed to acute type B hepatitis. *N Engl J Med* 293:1055, 1975.

Seeff LB. Type B hepatitis after needle-stick exposure: Prevention with hepatitis B immune globulin. *Ann Intern Med* 88:285, 1978.

9

Meningitis

The term meningitis is used for any state of inflammation of the linings of the brain and spinal cord. Such inflammation requires prompt diagnostic tests and, when indicated, treatment. Treatment may include precautions to prevent spread in the hospital, since certain types of meningitis are contagious. Although chemical agents, tumors, and trauma may inflame the meninges, the discussion in this chapter is restricted to infectious meningitis.

Infections of the central nervous system may be divided into those that affect the leptomeninges (meningitis) and those that involve neural tissue (encephalitis, myelitis, and radiculitis). The symptoms of each are related to the effects of the disease on the function of the involved part. The meninges are supportive structures that produce and absorb spinal fluid. Inflammation of them causes pain on motion, increased intracranial pressure, and signs of nerve entrapment. When infection disturbs neural tissue, there is a loss of integrative function: focal sensory or motor loss, acute intellectual defects, seizures, or altered consciousness.

In many cases, the disease syndromes of central nervous system infection overlap. Meningitis and encephalitis can be quite similar because of the intimate anatomical and vascular relationship between neurological tissue and its covering. Peripheral nerve infections, such as shingles (varicella zoster virus) can cause either meningitis, if the spinal nerve roots are involved, or encephalitis, if cranial nerves are affected, or a combination of both diseases.

Meningitis

Infection of the central nervous system can arise in a number of ways. The organism may be blood-borne and spread from remote infections; there may be a direct extension of infection from a contiguous locus along the peripheral nerve, as in a virus infection; or traumatic disruption of protective structures, such as a skull fracture, may permit direct introduction of the organism. Obviously, then, all classes of organisms—bacteria, fungi, parasites, and viruses—may infect the central nervous system.

Meningitis occurs as a sequela of some extraneural event. In children or adults, it may spread blood-borne from a remote locus, such as skin, lungs, urinary tract, or even the nasal sinuses. Surgery may introduce infection directly, and trauma may break a portal in skin, external ear canal, or nose to the CNS. In newborns, hematogenous meningitis is the rule, arising from aspiration of infected amniotic fluid, the GI tract, intravascular lines, or other life-support systems. Increased susceptibility to meningitis may accompany immune suppression, chronic disease, prematurity, or old age.

Some contagious forms of meningitis may spread within close groups. A case of meningococcemia in a family brings a ten-fold increased risk of meningococcal infection, including meningitis, for the other family members. Similar examples are detailed below.

As stated above, the diagnosis of meningitis does not necessarily indicate infection. Inflammation of the meninges may be caused by any irritating substance, such as chemicals, that contacts it, by tumors, and by inflammatory diseases, such as systemic lupus erythematosus. Central nervous system findings do not, however, always make it possible to distinguish viral from noninfectious meningitis. Viral meningitis is diagnosed by its acute onset and the absence of specific signs of tumor or other noninfectious disease. The majority of cases of bacterial meningitis are easily distinguished by cerebral spinal fluid findings and frequently the presence of a primary bacterial infection that has spread to the meninges. Though the history, physical examination, and pathophysiology are similar in different forms of meningitis, certain morphologic and epidemiologic clues suggest a specific etiology. Except for viral (18 percent) and certain forms of chronic meningitis (50 to 60 percent) a specific diagnosis can almost always be made within 24 to 72 hours.

Bacterial meningitis

Neisseria meningitidis (meningococcal meningitis) is the commonest cause of late winter and early spring meningitis in children and adolescents. It also appears in epidemic settings, such as summer camps and military basic training sites. The disease, referred to as cerebrospinal fever, epidemic meningitis, meningococcemia, and spotted fever, is usually associated with crowded living quarters. Onset is related to fatigue and overcrowding; it occurs more often among males than females.

Serogroups A, B, C, and Y are most often incriminated. Group A is the most common and presumably the most virulent, based on the observation that a rising frequency of nasopharyngeal carriers of group A is almost always followed by an increase in clinical meningitis. The bacteria are gram negative bean-shaped cocci, frequently seen within polymorphonuclear neutrophil leukocytes in stained preparations of cerebrospinal fluid. The organisms are quite sensitive to drying, ultraviolet light, and heat and must be rapidly placed in culture media if they are to grow. They grow best in a moist environment containing five percent CO_2.

Meningococci are carried in the nasopharynx. They are probably spread from person to person in crowded circumstances by droplets of respiratory secretion. Asymptomatic carriers may serve as reservoirs of infection. Fatigue seems to increase the rate of acquisition of the carrier state, as does intimate contact. Close contact, such as among household members or those with mouth-to-mouth contact, increases the risk of meningococcal infection in a given individual from the usual 1:1,000,000 per year to 1:10,000. An incubation period of three to four days is most common, though the range is two to 10 days.

There are three phases to the disease. In the colonization stage, the patient may be asymptomatic or have a mild upper respiratory infection, yet be a source of infection to others. In the second, septicemic stage, petechiae appear. These are usually generalized in infants, but in children and adults skin lesions are most often on the legs. They may be minute or confluent, even ecchymotic. Early in the second stage, petechiae may be so few that they can be detected only by careful examination. Phase three occurs with the characteristic clinical signs of meningitis: stiff neck, severe throbbing headache, fever, chills, backache, and vomiting. Death may occur within four hours of onset, particularly in the overwhelming septicemic form called Waterhouse-Friderichsen syndrome.

Avoiding direct or droplet contact with infected people is the main preventive measure. Patients should be put in respiratory isolation until 24 hours after effective therapy. Prophylactic treatment with the antibiotics rifampin or minocycline is recommended for family members of patients with meningococcal infection; their risk of becoming infected is several hundred times greater than that of casual contacts, such as hospital per-

Meningitis

sonnel. Because of the brief, relatively remote contact between patients and most hospital personnel, prophylaxis is not used except under rare circumstances. However, masks should be worn until 24 hours after treatment is begun to avoid inhaling infected droplets. Vaccine for types A and C may be used in epidemics.

Haemophilus influenzae is the most common cause of bacterial meningitis in children. Infants from six months to three years of age, who lack the protective antibody, are most susceptible. The syndrome is uncommon after age eight, but is sometimes seen in adults with underlying immunological defect or cerebrospinal fluid leak.

The organisms are pleomorphic gram negative rods that may be mistaken for pneumococci or meningococci in stained specimens. Six types are defined by capsular content, with type B the cause of 95 percent of the cases.

H. influenzae occupies the upper respiratory tract of infants and children and is transmitted person to person. It may rapidly colonize the occupants of a nursery, posing a potential threat of disease outbreak. Clinical illness may present as upper respiratory infection, such as epiglottitis or otitis media or pneumonia, and may progress to bacteremia and meningitis. Fever, sore throat, hoarseness, and barking cough are the clinical symptoms. The disease may progress to fulminant within hours.

The need for special precautions is undefined. Antibiotic prophylaxis of contacts is not recommended, except in epidemic circumstances in nurseries.

Streptococcus pneumoniae (pneumococcus) is the most common cause of bacterial meningitis, with peak incidence in children younger than one and adults older than 50. It occurs most often in infants with otitis media, mastoiditis, and pneumonia, and elderly alcoholics and those with pneumonia. In other age groups, infection is often associated with skull fractures; sickle cell disease is a predisposing factor at any age. Mortality remains high—at 35 to 40 percent—despite availability of effective antibiotics.

The organisms are lancet-shaped gram positive diplococci and grow rapidly on blood agar in an environment of five percent CO_2. Pneumococci are typed by their polysaccharide capsule. Type III organisms, which possess thick capsules, are the most virulent. Pneumococci become part of the normal flora of the throats of many persons during the spring and fall months. They are presumably spread by direct contact and droplets. Because of their sensitivity to drying in coughed secretions and the high prevalence of carriers in the absence of frank clinical disease, special isolation precautions are not employed for patients with pneumococcal meningitis. Antibiotic prophylaxis of contacts is not used. Pneumococcal vaccine, however, especially in those at highest risk, may be useful.

Escherichia coli is the most common cause of meningitis in the newborn. Organisms are gram negative rods. A specific capsular antigen (K1), similar to that of group B in meningococcus, may play a role in virulence. Organisms may be acquired from the maternal birth canal or nursery personnel who may be carriers. Because of the impracticality of screening all personnel and mothers for K1 positive *E. coli*, special precautions are not routinely practiced. The organisms persist as part of the normal fecal flora of many adults. Infected neonates are isolated in an incubator for 24 to 48 hours until the organism is identified.

Other bacteria that occasionally cause meningitis include *Streptococcus pyogenes* (groups A and B), *Staphylococcus aureus, Listeria monocytogenes, Klebsiella pneumoniae, Salmonella, Flavobacterium,* and *Mycobacterium tuberculosis.* The gram positive chains of cocci of *Streptococcus pyogenes* can be found in small numbers in the respiratory, GI, and genital tracts. Fetal infection can occur as the result of aspirating contaminated amniotic fluid. Infection in the neonate may result from colonization in the birth canal. Group B streptococcal meningitis is the second most common form of neonatal meningitis. It may complicate septicemia or pneumonia. Septicemia is the principal presentation in the first two days of life, but pneumonia is commoner later, after day 4 or 5. This suggests two sources of colonization for the neonate, the mother's birth canal and hospital employees. In older children and adults, antecedent infection is the usual cause. Transmission is by direct contact or droplet. Isolation is used until 24 hours following effective therapy.

Staphylococcus aureus and the related *Staphylococcus epidermidis* are rarely causes of meningitis, except in three circumstances: infective endocarditis, spread from adjacent osteomyelitis, and after neurosurgery. Diagnosis is difficult sometimes, because staphylococci may be introduced into CSF as contaminants during specimen collection. In the hospital, patients acquire staphylococcal meningitis as complications from their own skin, hands of personnel, or, rarely, contaminated instruments. Isolation, except in the presence of draining wounds or pneumonia, is unnecessary.

Epidemics of *Klebsiella pneumoniae* are common in large neurosurgical units. The organism is a gram negative, plump, encapsulated bacillus which is part of the fecal flora of humans and animals. They can be typed by capsular antisera, which is useful for tracing epidemics. *Klebsi-*

ella persist in neurosurgical units because of their facility in developing antibiotic resistance and widespread antibiotic prophylaxis.

Listeria monocytogenes, easily mistaken for diphtheroids, cause infections most often in neonates and immune-suppressed patients. Isolation is not required. The principal reservoir in man is the genital tract.

The nontyphoid *Salmonella* exist in nature as gram negative bacilli, normally resident in animals and animal feed. They are most often acquired from contaminated food, occasionally water. Typing into groups A to E is done for epidemiologic purposes. They rarely cause meningitis, but when they do, it is most often in children, individuals with sickle cell disease, and the immune-suppressed.

Flavobacterium, a gram negative bacillus that produces a yellow pigment in culture, is a common contaminant of water. It is occasionally transmitted in aerosols, such as respiratory therapy equipment, and may cause meningitis in ICU patients.

A gram negative comma-shaped bacillus, *Pseudomonas* is classified into several species. The most common, *P. aeruginosa,* is an inhabitant of casual water—drinking water, sink drains, unused irrigating fluids, and the like—and, because of its ubiquitous distribution and potential for antibiotic resistance, has become a major hospital pathogen. It rarely spreads to the normal intact meninges, but causes meningitis after being introduced by trauma or neurosurgery.

In stained specimens, *Mycobacterium tuberculosis* is acid-fast (retains specific stains despite acid-alcohol decolorizing) and stains with certain fluorescent dyes. It grows slowly on specially prepared media and requires up to six weeks for identification. It is spread from person to person from pulmonary loci by coughing (droplets). Patients with isolated meningitis and no lung infection thus require no precautions, but associated cavitary pulmonary disease dictates respiratory isolation of the patient. Clinical recognition of this meningitis may be delayed because of its similarity to fungal or viral meningitis. See Chapter 11 for a fuller discussion of tuberculosis.

Viral meningitis

Of the 18 percent of cases of aseptic meningitis with confirmed etiologies, 15 percent are due to enteroviruses. These include the coxsackie-, echo-, and polioviruses. These are all small (pico), RNA-containing viruses that belong to the picornavirus family. All have the potential of causing encephalitis as well as meningitis and all are natural inhabitants of the alimentary tract, gaining access to the central nervous system via the bloodstream or along neural tracts (poliomyelitis). All are resistant to acid, thus their infectivity for the lower tract is preserved after swallowing, despite passage through the stomach. All appear in the stool of infected individuals and enteric precautions are employed, as well as secretion precautions.

Enteroviruses are carried in the alimentary tracts of many asymptomatic individuals. They are excreted in feces and, when they appear in abundance in sewage, they may contaminate wells, pools, streams, and drinking water supplies. Their levels in sewage and streams correlate well with the prevalence of infection in a community. Infections peak in spring, summer, and fall, related to increased outdoor activity and consequent water contamination. Some reports trace outbreaks among adults to day-care centers. Young children frequently have mild or asymptomatic infection. Parents and older siblings acquire the illness from them after they contract it from other children at the centers.

Invasion of the central nervous system may occur as a complication of mumps, with sequelae ranging from mild meningeal irritation to more severe encephalitis. Mumps virus (*Myxovirus parotitis*) is so named because of its lipid-containing, ether-sensitive outer membrane and its predilection to infection of the parotid glands. There are no known animal reservoirs or nonhuman vectors. Mumps is exclusively a human disease and appears primarily in children. Infection spreads via microdroplets of saliva. Salivary secretions are infectious for several days during incubation of the disease, and from asymptomatic infected persons.

Mumps virus may cause aseptic meningitis (two percent of etiologically identified cases), meningoencephalitis, and is the most common cause of viral encephalitis in the U.S., accounting for 12 to 25 percent of cases. The virus initially infects the secretory cells of the upper respiratory tract. Respiratory precautions are employed for patients with mumps.

Lymphocytic choriomeningitis virus (LCM), a member of the arenavirus family, has an RNA core and a lipid-sensitive coat. It is related to the notorious Lassa virus. Its natural host is wild mice. In their colonies it is passed in utero from mother to fetus. Pet hamsters, guinea pigs, dogs, monkeys, and swine have also been implicated in transmitting the virus. It is excreted in the saliva, urine, feces, and semen of infected animals.

Infections occur in laboratory workers throughout the year and in others in fall months when rodents migrate into homes from the fields. The disease has a wide spectrum of clinical manifestations that may range from flu-like symptoms to hemorrhagic meningoencephalitis. The latter occurs rarely in man. Person-to-person transmission is rare. Isolation is not practiced.

Meningitis

The herpesviruses (*Herpesvirus hominus,* varicella zoster, Epstein-Barr) are all DNA viruses that can infect human epithelial cells. All may cause meningitis, radiculitis, meningoencephalitis, and viral encephalitis. Of the three, herpesvirus is the most common cause of aseptic meningitis and presumably gains access to the meninges via hematogenous spread. In women, and to a lesser extent in men, primary genital herpes frequently ascends the nerve roots or travels the bloodstream to cause a self-limited aseptic meningitis. Recurrences may accompany cutaneous exacerbation.

Varicella zoster virus is suspected of reaching the meninges via neural axons. Meningitis is rare in infectious mononucleosis (EB virus). Other causes of viral meningitis include measles virus, encephalomyocarditis virus, hepatitis virus, adenoviruses 1, 2, 5, 6, and 7, and rhinovirus.

Fungal meningitis

The commonest fungal cause of meningitis is *Cryptococcus neoformans,* an encapsulated yeast-like organism. Twelve species of cryptococcus have been identified, but only *C. neoformans* is pathogenic for man. When freshly isolated from the spinal fluid, the organism has a thick capsule and reproduces by budding. It produces urease, permitting it to be distinguished from *Candida* in the laboratory. The human pathogen grows well at 37°C, whereas saprophytic species require lower temperatures in order to grow.

The organisms may be found worldwide, growing in most shady soil enriched with avian feces; growth is particularly common in pigeon droppings. The disease is probably caused by inhalation of dust contaminated by living fungus. Laboratory and human-to-human transmission has not been documented. The immunosuppressed and the high-risk patients (alcoholics, diabetics) are more prone to develop the disease. However, many individuals with no underlying problems are found to have cryptococcosis. This disease may range from a mild pulmonary illness to chronic meningitis (lasting longer than three weeks) and indeed has a predilection for the central nervous system. Isolation is not necessary, as person-to-person transmission has not been observed.

Coccidioides immitis (valley fever) is a fungus common to the Southwestern United States, Mexico, and South America. It is present in desert soils and grows as thick-walled spherules containing several hundred endospores. Filamentous mycelial forms also grow in the soil. These may fragment and release air-borne arthrospores that are highly infectious if inhaled. Thus cultures of *C. immitis,* which contain primarily mycelia, must be carefully handled in the laboratory.

Since the tissue form is predominantly spherules, person-to-person transmission is unlikely and isolation unnecessary. The disease in the lungs may vary from localized pneumonitis to chronic cavity disease that resembles tuberculosis. Dissemination from the lungs may reach any tissue of the body and leptomeninges are frequently involved.

Histoplasma capsulatum, a yeast in infected tissues, normally causes an acute, self-limited infection in humans. From its source in bird excreta, principally of starlings and chickens, it may be inhaled into the lungs. In very rare cases, it causes progressive, usually fatal disease, including meningitis. Isolation is not used. Person-to-person transmission occurs rarely from skin lesions.

Blastomyces dermatitidis is a yeast in tissues, but a mold on laboratory medium. It causes skin, bone, and lung lesions, and rarely may disseminate to the meninges. The source of the fungus in nature is unknown, and person-to-person transmission does not ordinarily occur, except by direct contact. Skin and wound precautions are used for skin lesions.

Candida species, predominantly *C. albicans,* may rarely disseminate to the meninges, particularly in diabetics and cancer patients. They are normal inhabitants of the human gastrointestinal tract and oropharynx, but may become invasive after immunosuppression or broad-spectrum antibiotic therapy or in diabetics. The common determinant of invasion appears to be increased available glucose for growth. *C. albicans* and *C. tropicalis* are the most invasive because of their capacity to form phagocyte-resistant mycelia in vivo. Isolation is not used as *Candida* are part of most persons' upper respiratory flora.

Protozoa

Toxoplasma gondii, a protozoon, causes one of the commonest infections of man. Sources in nature include feline feces and raw meat. The feline species is the only one shedding fecal oocysts and is apparently the definitive host. However, since all mammals may be infected, carnivores, such as man, may be infected by eating cyst-bearing raw or undercooked meat. Isolated meningitis is rarely seen, but meningoencephalitis, especially in the immunodeficient host, is not uncommon. Isolation is not employed.

Naeglaria and *Acanthamoeba,* free-living fresh-water amebae, may rarely cause meningitis in water skiers or divers who presumably acquire infection through minor fractures of the cribriform plate. The disease has been fatal to all but a few of the rare individuals reported to have acquired it. *(Text continued on page 100)*

Meningitis

Table 9-1

Nonbacterial meningitis

Etiology	Diagnostic aids	Age	Incubation
Enterovirus	Viral studies on CSF, blood, feces, pharynx, urine; CSF analysis; sharp rise in summer	Most common in young children and young adults	3-8 days
LCM	Viral studies on blood, urine, CSF, nasopharynx; most common in winter and spring	All ages; young adults most common	8-13 days; 15-21 days for meningitis
Mumps	Viral studies on CSF and parotid duct secretions; most common in winter and early spring	Most common in childhood	12-26 days
Cryptococcus	History of underlying disease; history of exposure; culture of CSF, urine, sputum, sinus drainage; latex agglutination of CSF, serum, and urine most valuable	Mostly adults	Unknown
Coccidioides	Smear and culture of CSF and sputum; skin test, precipitin, and complement-fixation or serology	All ages, but more than half of patients are in the 15- to 20-year age bracket	1-4 weeks
Histoplasma	Smear, stain, and culture: ulcer exudates, sputum, blood, bone marrow; biopsy specimens; serology for serum antibody.	All ages, but more frequently in adults, middle-aged, and old men	5-18 days

(cont'd)_____

Signs and symptoms	Therapy	Prevention
Fever, headache, muscle stiffness, paralysis (1-2% polio) diarrhea, pharyngitis, cough, myalgia, photophobia	Bed rest, analgesics; maintain fluid and electrolyte balance; physical therapy when required; excretion precautions	Vaccine (polio); improve personal hygiene and sanitation practices
Depends on the area involved and severity of the lesion; may range from mild meningeal irritation to coma from meningoencephalitis	None, except to treat specific symptoms; maintain fluid, electrolyte balance; provide respiratory assistance	Good sanitation; rodent control—surveillance of mice and hamster breeding areas
Fever, headache, lethargy, nausea and vomiting, stiff neck; Kernig's and Brudzinski's signs may be absent	Aspirin for pain and fever; maintain fluid and electrolyte balance; respiratory precautions	Vaccine any time after one year of age; vaccine administered at time of exposure is of questionable value; mumps hyperimmunoglobulin is also of questionable value but should be considered for the immunosuppressed individual who should not be given the vaccine
Chronic course: headache increases in intensity and frequency; changes in ventilation, motor function, cranial nerve function	Amphotericin B in conjunction with flucytosine	Unknown
Persistent fever, headache, and toxicity following pulmonary infection	Amphotericin B	Avoid exposure to contaminated dust
Chronic headache, confusion, fever, stiff neck	Surgery to relieve intracranial pressure; amphotericin B	Surveillance of chicken breeding coops; avoid unnecessary exposure to same

Meningitis

Susceptible hosts and pathogenesis

Most episodes of meningitis occur in hosts with normal defenses, and are therefore attributable to pathogenic characteristics of the infecting organisms. However, immunocompromised hosts have, in addition to the common bacterial and viral meningitides, a profusion of uncommon infections. In general, decreased humoral immunity leads only to an increased incidence of the common forms of bacterial meningitis, but decreased cellular immunity may be associated with listerial, mycobacterial, fungal, or parasitic meningitis, as resistance to these appears to depend primarily on elements of the cellular immune system.

Invasion of the meninges occurs via several pathways—direct inoculation, hematogenous from remote or proximal foci, and along nerve fibers. Direct inoculation may occur during lumbar puncture, neurosurgical procedures, or after traumatic fracture of a part of the bony covering of the CNS. Organisms include those that inhabit the body at the point of trauma or the traumatic instrument.

Hematogenous spread from the point of invasion is most common. Thus pneumococci spread from lungs, middle ears, or sinuses, *H. influenzae* from upper respiratory tract, and meningococci from the nasopharynx. Cryptococci and fungi generally spread from a primary lung focus, but *Candida* may be inoculated directly into the bloodstream from intravenous sets.

Such viruses as polio and herpes may spread along peripheral nerves, but others, such as coxsackievirus and even occasionally genital herpes, invade the bloodstream and, from there, the meninges. When meningitis occurs repetitively one should suspect a fistula, such as a fractured cribriform plate, petrus ridge, or congenital defect.

The precise factors contributing to localization of pneumococci, meningococci, *H. influenzae,* cryptococci, and coccidioides on the meninges are unknown, but it is clear that bloodstream invasion with these organisms carries a far greater risk of meningitis than with most other organisms. Specific hairlike bacterial surface organelles (pili) may determine adhesiveness of certain bacteria to the linings of meningeal blood vessels.

The acute local reaction to meningeal infection is with polymorphonuclear leukocytes. However, whereas the number of PMNs increases with most bacterial meningitis with time, the response shifts to lymphocytes early in the course of most nonbacterial forms of meningitis. Locally, glial (neural inflammatory) cells may also participate in the meningeal reaction. All forms of meningeal irritation may provoke exudation, increasing spinal-fluid proteins. Certain forms evoke specific antibody formation by plasma cells in the CNS, with increases in CSF globulin content. Bacterial and fungal meningitis can interfere with active transport of glucose into and out of the CSF, with resultant hypoglycorrhachia (low CSF glucose). Viruses, except for mumps and lymphocytic choriomeningitis virus (LCM), rarely cause this phenomenon.

Symptomatology

Symptoms of meningitis vary with the class of causative agent and may provide useful clues in diagnosis. Bacterial meningitis symptoms are those of the infection and of increased CSF pressure. Rigors, fever, malaise, and headache predominate. In infants, stupor progressing to coma and flaccidity are common, whereas in older children and adults bursting headache, stiffness of the paraspinous muscles, and hyperactive deep tendon reflexes are common. Vomiting, tinnitus, vertigo, diplopia, seizures, and delirium are common. In viral meningitis, systemic symptoms such as diarrhea, myalgia, pharyngitis, cough, photophobia, and retroorbital pain accompany the fever, headache, and stiff neck and are helpful in distinguishing bacterial from viral meningitis.

Clinical, laboratory, and X-ray findings

Clinical findings vary with age of the host and infecting organisms. Profound nuchal rigidity occurs with most bacterial and viral meningitis in adults, but flaccidity predominates in infants. Bulging of the fontanelles in infants often proclaims increased intracranial pressure, but dehydration from vomiting and diarrhea may mask the sign. Delirium early in the course, progressing to stupor and coma, is common with bacterial meningitis, but uncommon in viral. Examination of the ocular fundi frequently reveals papilledema (swelling of the optic nerve), and function of cranial nerves may be altered because of increased intracranial pressure. Since viral meningitis most often accompanies extraneural virus infection, the extraneural signs (adenopathy, pharyngitis, skin lesions) may be prominent. Fungal and tuberculous meningitis may mimic CNS tumors, with focal neurologic defects and slowly changing sensorium. Toxoplasmosis can be confused with infectious mononucleosis, cytomegalovirus infection, or lymphoma.

The peripheral white count is usually high in bacterial meningitis, but is normal or low in other forms. Urinalysis may reveal an inappropriately concentrated urine (inappropriate antidiuretic hormone syndrome) or signs of bacteriuria in gram negative bacterial meningitis. The spinal fluid examination provides the key to diagnosis, with gram stain, culture, cell count, protein, and sugar determinations essential components of the examination. In hemophilus, pneumococcus, *E. coli,* meningococcus, and cryptococcus meningitis, determination of antigens of the infecting organism in CSF by counterimmunoelectrophoresis or agglutination reaction can give a specific diagnosis in minutes. Culture of spinal fluid should be from fresh whole CSF and centrifuged sediment. Cultures should be immediately inoculated onto warmed blood agar, EMB, Löwenstein-Jensen, and Sabouraud's selective and nonselective agar. Blood agar plates should be incubated in five percent CO_2. If findings suggest viral meningitis, blood for acute phase viral antibody titers should be collected immediately, and again two to three weeks later. Stool for viral culture should also be collected.

Gram stains of CSF are essential, but debris and precipitated stain may confuse interpretation. Practice in interpretation of gram stains improves performance. CSF placed in an incubator overnight at 37°C will frequently show bacteria on gram stain or AFB stain, due to growth of the organisms. Cultures of potential primary sources of infection (nasopharynx, sputum, ears, blood) should be collected before treatment is begun.

Differential diagnosis

These are to be considered in differential diagnosis: Metastatic tumors to the meninges, CNS leukemia, CNS lupus erythematosus or other vasculitis, embolic meningitis from infectious endocarditis, infected parameningeal focus (otitis media, subdural or epidural abscess, paranasal sinusitis, brain abscess, venous sinus septic phlebitis).

Prognosis

Various complications may follow meningitis. These include cranial nerve palsies, blindness, deafness, motor or intellectual defects, hydrocephalus, abscess, subdural effusion, and death.

Death occurs in up to 100 percent of patients with untreated bacterial meningitis. However, it is rare with viral and tuberculous meningitis. Despite vigorous therapy, at least 20 percent of patients with fungal meningitis die. Mortality from treated bacterial meningitis occurs most commonly in the very young and very old, 100 percent of infants with *Pseudomonas* meningitis being reported to succumb, 70 percent with enterobacterial gram negative meningitis, and 25 to 50 percent of others. Recent reports of novel forms of antibiotic treatment suggest that these results may be significantly improved. Most forms of bacillary meningitis have 50 percent mortality in the treated aged, except for *H. influenzae* (10 percent) and *N. meningitidis* (25 percent).

Infants with meningitis may not manifest overt motor or intellectual defects for up to several years after recovery, so that data on prognosis are incomplete.

Medical treatment

The goals of medical treatment of meningitis are two: to sterilize the CSF and meningeal foci and to prevent sequelae due to inflammation.

Most antimicrobial drugs achieve low concentrations in the CSF, due to the relative impermeability of the blood-CSF or blood-brain barrier. Even when inflammation disrupts the barrier, CSF antimicrobial concentrations generally are 10 percent or less of simultaneous blood concentrations. Thus, large doses of IV antimicrobials at frequent intervals are required, and often intrathecal or intraventricular drug administration is necessary. In desperate circumstances, large doses of parenteral corticosteroids may reduce inflammation in the meninges and cerebral edema and thus be of some therapeutic value.

Fluids should be carefully restricted, as retention due to inappropriate antidiuretic hormone activity frequently complicates infectious meningitis and may lead to fulminant fatal cerebral edema.

Bibliography

Benenson AS, ed. *Control of Communicable Diseases in Man* (13th ed). Washington DC: American Public Health Association, 1981.

Davis BD. *Microbiology.* Hagerstown Md: Harper & Row, 1980.

Hoeprich PD, ed. *Infectious Diseases* (2nd ed). Hagerstown Md: Harper & Row, 1977.

Krugman S. *Infectious Diseases of Children* (7th ed). St Louis: Mosby, 1980.

Remington JS and Klein JO, eds. *Infectious Diseases of the Fetus and Newborn Infant.* Philadelphia: Saunders, 1976.

Top FH and Wehrle PF, eds. *Communicable and Infectious Diseases* (8th ed). St Louis: Mosby, 1976.

Youmans GP, Paterson PY, Sommers HM, eds. *The Biologic and Clinical Basis of Infectious Diseases* (2nd ed). Philadelphia: Saunders, 1980.

10

Scabies and pediculosis

Since 1972 or 1973, there has been a worldwide epidemic of scabies. The reason for this is unknown. It is of interest that in the late 1960s the frequency of scabies among pets, particularly household dogs, increased dramatically. The relationship between this and the human outbreak is not understood, however, since the dog scabies, a variety of *Sarcoptes scabiei,* causes only temporary infestation in humans. The epidemic of scabies has afflicted rich and poor, clean and dirty, old and young, men and women equally. Current clinical presentations vary considerably from that described in older textbooks, making diagnosis difficult. Also today, treatment, previously accomplished with a single application of scabicide, usually has to be extended to two or three applications.

Of particular concern to health-care workers is the occurrence of scabies among nursing-home residents and hospitalized patients. Many cases of transmission from patients to hospital workers and vice versa have been reported. The best protection against scabies outbreaks is prompt recognition and treatment of index cases.

Causative organism

The mite that causes scabies is formally designated *Sarcoptes scabiei var. hominis.* The female form is oval, flat, and approximately 0.4 mm long.

The mite has four pairs of legs on which it moves rather rapidly, approximately 2.5 cm, or one inch, per minute. The male mite is longer, approximately 1.5 mm long. The sexual forms differ in their behavior on the skin. The female travels across the skin until it finds a favorable spot and burrows beneath the outer layer of skin to the stratum granulosum, where it begins to lay eggs. The male mite largely stays on the surface and only occasionally enters a burrow for food or to copulate with a female mite. The females, because of their burrowing, are responsible for the symptoms of scabies, but because they stay largely beneath the surface of the skin, they are not easily transmitted.

Prolonged intimate contact between individuals is most likely to result in spread of disease. In young sexually promiscuous individuals, scabies behaves as a venereal disease. In one VD clinic, more than two percent of patients seen presented with symptoms of scabies. Because of this, it is important to assess young sexually active individuals who have scabies for the presence of other sexually transmitted diseases.

Epidemiology

Classically, scabies was seldom seen in individuals with good hygiene. It was most frequently seen in military combat groups, prisons, and people living in poverty. But the more recent epidemic has not respected classic descriptions. Organisms may survive at room temperature for several days in clothing, but Mellanby's studies for the British Ministry of Health 30 years ago clearly demonstrated that clothing and bedclothes are not a major source of scabies. In these studies, Mellanby had experimental subjects wear undergarments of persons with scabies and sleep in their unwashed sheets. The result was that fewer than two in 100 individuals so exposed developed any sign of scabies. The mites are killed within 10 minutes at a temperature of 50°C, a temperature commonly achieved in commercial and many home water heaters. Casual contact is likewise unlikely to spread the disease, unless the afflicted areas on the patient are heavily excoriated, exposing the mites so that they can be transmitted promptly. Scabies tends to occur in clusters within family groups or other contexts in which intimate person-to-person contacts occur.

Pathogenesis

Infestation begins when the fertilized female burrows beneath the skin in such areas as the creases between the fingers and lays large eggs in the burrows, one to two daily, for her entire life span of four to five weeks. These eggs hatch after several days and go through two nymph stages, requiring approximately 11 days, to become young adults. These adults then migrate to meet their opposite sexual number, copulate, and repeat the cycle.

The initial stages of primary scabies in a human cause few or no symptoms or signs. Indeed, the incubation period is generally four to six weeks. As the individual acquires sensitivity to the proteins of the mite, allergy develops, itching and rash appear, and symptoms become florid. With repeated exposure of a person previously infested and sensitized, the incubation period can be as short as one to two days. Clinical illness can be perpetuated indefinitely, although, under most circumstances, the infestation spontaneously terminates in one to two months. The number of female mites per infested person is usually 11.

Infection manifestation

The burrows caused by the mite are classically found in the lateral aspects and creases between the fingers, the flexor surface of the wrist, the extensor surface of the elbow, the areole of the breasts, the groin, and the creases beneath the buttocks. In adults, the face and scalp are rarely, if ever, affected. This is probably due to the maturity of sebaceous glands in those areas; presumably, the sebum immobilizes or kills the mites. However, in children with immature sebaceous glands, the face and scalp may be involved.

The recent epidemic is interesting in that in more than 10 percent of individuals the organisms do not cause burrows and lesions are therefore atypical. When it is present, the burrow appears as a short, wavy, dirty-appearing line. At the distal end is a tiny blister. Approximately 0.5 mm proximal to the blister is the site where the female mite can be found.

The principal symptom of scabies is intense itching that occurs nocturnally and in most individuals is sufficiently severe to prevent sleep. This itching leads to vigorous scratching, and the areas scratched become secondarily infected, further confusing the diagnosis.

Diagnosis

With a good light and a hand lens magnifying four to five times, you can generally spot the mite as a black dot in the skin lesion. Using a scalpel blade, one can shave the top off the burrow and lift the mite out onto a microscope slide for confirmation. An alternative is to extract the mite from the burrow with a syringe and needle, but this takes some practice. Many health-care workers first place a drop of mineral oil over the mite to make sure that when it is lifted out of the burrow, the mite and the associated eggs are not flicked off the blade into the air and lost. If placed on a second drop of mineral oil on the slide, they can be easily observed. Using potassium hydroxide to clear the skin makes visualization of the mite easier, but dissolves eggs and fecal pellets, which are 30 to 40 times more numerous than the insects themselves.

Clinical forms of scabies

Scabies may take a variety of clinical forms, depending on the intensity of infestation, age of the patient, associated medication, and socioeconomic status. In clean individuals who develop scabies, the findings are frequently minimal. Lotions and other topicals are used abundantly in areas with itching, thus disguising the lesions. Burrows are hard to find, and a careful search is necessary. If an individual with itchy skin is given topical steroid creams to use, these may mask the signs and symptoms, leading to scabies incognito. Steroids may entirely mask the signs and symptoms, but they do not cure the infestation or alter transmission of the disease.

Nodular scabies occurs frequently in infants, but may occur at any age. Covered areas of the body are most frequently involved, particularly the male genitalia, groin, axillary region, and the beltline. Mites are seldom identified in the reddish brown pruritic nodules that develop. These nodules tend to persist, despite effective treatment, and are probably due to hypersensitivity. They clear spontaneously, but their clearing may be hastened by careful local injection of steroid solution. In infants and young children, misdiagnosis of scabies is frequent because burrows are generally not present, suspicion of scabies is less likely, and other conditions are frequently mimicked. The lesions may be nodular or vesicular. Vesicles may enlarge to form bullae filled with clear fluid. They are distributed atypically, and frequently involve the head, neck, palms, and soles of the feet. Secondary infection is common.

The most extensive form of scabies is so-called "Norwegian," or crusted, scabies. This form is rare, but it is highly contagious because of the extensive excoriation leading to surface-dwelling mites and heavy infestation. Norwegian scabies is generally present for an extensive period before diagnosis is made. It is therefore more commonly seen in the chronically ill, particularly in the mentally retarded and physically and immunologically debilitated patients, and seldom occurs in normal healthy individuals. The lesions are generally crusting areas of dermatosis of the hands and feet with deformation of the nails and red generalized scaling eruptions. Curiously, itching is not a prominent symptom.

Other forms of scabies include scabies in the bedridden, occurring in sites that are in constant contact with sheets, and scabies with other sexually-transmitted diseases, such as syphilis. Animal-transmitted scabies are self-limiting forms of infestation with animal-adapted species that lack the ability to burrow beneath the skin extensively and are unable to copulate in human skin.

Prevention

Prevention of scabies can be accomplished with effective isolation techniques for patients and personnel. Patients with a clinical diagnosis of scabies should be placed under wound and skin precautions until they have been under effective treatment for 24 hours. Second treatments are frequently necessary to make certain all eggs are destroyed. Personnel who are diagnosed as having scabies should not have patient contact until they have had 24 hours of successful treatment.

Personnel exposed to an infected person should receive preventive therapy on an individual basis. Those who have prolonged intimate contact, such as physical therapists who may be required to hold a patient close to their exposed skin for long periods, may benefit from preventive therapy. However, casual contact, such as that involved in routine physical examinations or brief nursing tasks, is not an indication for prophylaxis. Bed clothing and apparel should be washed in hot water and/or dried on hot cycle. Alternatively, these may be placed in sealed plastic bags for 10 or more days.

Medications

Four different medications are effective against scabies. The most commonly used, lindane, is reasonably safe for adults. Remember, however, that up to 10 percent of the drug spread on the skin subsequently appears in the urine, so absorption through the skin is considerable. This is of importance in children in whom excessive use of the drug has been known to cause CNS disorders including seizures. Lindane induces generalized seizures in the mite, with subsequent death.

Crotamiton is an alternative drug, which seems to be safe for children. Though some dermatologists feel that it is slightly less effective than lindane, comparative trials have not been published, and for most people the drug is effective. Precipitated sulfur is the oldest effective treatment in constant use. It is perfectly safe for infants and children but aesthetically less desirable. In addition, it requires three daily applications. Pyrethrins are newer scabicides that are infrequently employed.

Treatment procedure

Most treatment failures are due to failure of patients to completely carry out instructions. For example, crotamiton needs to be applied twice over a 24-hour interval and left in place for a total of 48 hours before bathing—directions with which many patients do not comply. Other directions on using the medication, especially in pregnancy, are to be followed carefully.

Close family contacts, particularly those that share the same bed with the patient, should have preventive treatment. Following treatment, symptoms may persist for up to four to six weeks. This should not cause alarm; it is not due to continued infestation, but to allergy to dead mites and eggs. These symptoms may be controlled with antihistamines or judicious use of steroid medication. With cases of reinfection, an antihistamine may be added for four or five days.

A variety of special instructions can be given to household members of patients with scabies. Obviously, they should avoid direct skin contact with infected areas of the patient until treatment is completed. They should also avoid contact with soiled linen and towels, although unnecessary fear of this should be discouraged. Soiled clothing and linens should be thoroughly laundered. A mattress upon which the patient has slept may be safely decontaminated by enclosing it in an airtight plastic bag for 10 days. A gamma benzene hexachloride spray can be used before enclosing.

An invariable consequence of scabies is excessive fear. The term for this disorder is acarophobia, which is a form of parasitosis delusion. Such patients present themselves over and over again with symptoms of scabies but no clinical signs and no diagnosable infestation. The individuals may benefit from psychiatric attention. In addition, guilt and shame are not infrequent in patients who develop scabies because of the known association of the disorder with poor personal hygiene and sexual promiscuity. Therefore, extensive patient education and reassurance are essential components of proper medical care.

Pediculosis

In 1970, there was a sharp increase in number of questions concerning pediculosis reaching the Centers for Disease Control in Atlanta. This coincided closely with the ban on DDT. Although there is no direct evidence that the two events are causally related, it is certainly true that epidemics of lice in the past were effectively controlled by mass treatment of residences and persons with DDT powder.

The current wave of pediculosis is affecting individuals at every socio-economic level. As in the past, pediculosis capitis (infestation of the head) is most commonly found in schoolchildren, but rarely in black children. Pubic lice (*Phthirus pubis*) are found most frequently in sexually active individuals. The highest incidence in women is in the 15 to 20 year age group, but in men most cases appear in patients older than age 20. Pediculosis corporis (infestation of the body), has remained stable in rates of occurrence, largely because it is restricted to circumstances of poor body hygiene and poverty. It is fortunate that the occurrence of body lice is so restricted, because this is the only form of human louse that transmits systemic disease.

Causative organisms

The organisms of head lice and body lice have a great deal of morphologic similarity and can interbreed, which suggests a common evolutionary past. Some speculate that when man began to wear clothing, head lice migrated to the body and adapted to a new, safe residence. The *Pediculus capitis* and *Pediculus corporis* are both elongated, six-legged organisms with long abdominal segments. The crab louse (*Phthirus pubis*) is a broad, flat organism with large, powerful claw-like legs, which are well-adapted to grasping the widely spaced hairs in the pubic region.

The eggs of pubic and head lice are laid at the point where a hair shaft joins the skin. They are oval, white, and adhere tightly to the hair. Over the seven to 10 days required for the egg to mature, the hair grows approximately one-fourth of an inch, so that eggs found greater than that distance from the skin are unlikely to still contain lice. The eggs of body lice are laid in seams of clothing. The body louse moves much more rapidly than the head or pubic louse and leaves the seams in warm areas, such as the axilla or groin, to travel over the skin for feeding purposes. Only in heavy infestations are you likely to find eggs or lice on the body of the person with body lice.

Epidemiology

Head and pubic lice will spread despite a high level of cleanliness. Spread is most often by direct contact, although fomites such as combs, shared clothing, or bedclothes can be vehicles for transmission. Head lice are most often acquired by schoolchildren who share combs, hats, and frequently lie down on furniture or carpets in close proximity to one another. Pubic lice tend to infect young adults. They are spread most often through sexual contact, although children can acquire them from close contact with infested parents. The lice frequently harbor in the eyebrows and eyelashes of the affected children. Body lice are spread in circumstances of poor personal hygiene and are most often found in patients in public hospitals, thus the name "vagabond's disease." Body lice are rather rare in the United States. They can transmit epidemic typhus, trench fever, and a variety of relapsing fever (Borellia).

Pathogenesis

The eggs of body lice laid in seams of clothing go through maturation, hatching, and a series of nymph forms to reach adult form in approximately three weeks. Each louse has a life span of approximately one month, and during this time the female can produce as many as 300 eggs. Body lice migrate onto the body of the infested individual to feed, leaving behind a telltale red papule.

Head and pubic lice lay their eggs on hair shafts. They mature and hatch in approximately one week. The young lice go through a series of moults to reach maturity. Head lice survive approximately one month and pubic lice about 15 days. There is some difference of opinion about the ability of lice to survive separated from the human host. Head and pubic lice will not survive more than 48 hours without the warmth and blood meals of the human body and will die from starvation. Body lice are probably also dependent on blood meals, although some investigators believe they can survive up to seven days. The eggs of all forms of lice can survive off the human body but after seven days will probably not hatch, even if they are again placed in a circumstance where body warmth provides the proper environment.

Signs, symptoms, and diagnosis

Early infestation with lice is difficult to detect. The nits are close to the skin and are not easily visible. Itching, a cardinal symptom, does not occur until the patient develops hypersensitivity; therefore, the infested person has generally borne the lice for well over a month before nits or itching become apparent. In pediculosis capitis, the white, glistening, empty eggs of the lice firmly attached to the hair are easily seen in the sunlight. These must be distinguished from skin scales and dandruff, which are not very difficult to remove from the hair. To establish a diagnosis, one can comb hair with a very-fine-tooth comb over a dark surface or onto a glass slide. Under a microscope or magnifying glass, the eggs appear as oval, hollow structures firmly adhering to the hair. Associated itching may cause the patient to scratch vigorously and lead to secondary infection with pyoderma and regional enlargement of lymph nodes.

Patients with body lice frequently have numerous vertical excoriations due to intense itching. These are often bacterially infected. Lice are not commonly found on the body except in individuals with heavy infestations. A more likely place to find them is on the seams of clothing, particularly the armpits, the beltline, the collar, and the groin region. Eggs may also be found in these areas. The lice are easiest to identify after they have fed, when they take on a reddish brown color. A characteristic manifestation of body lice in children, sleek grey spots that appear on the extremities and fade over the course of a few hours, is seen in only about 10 percent of those infested.

The organisms of pubic lice are distinctive in their appearance. Like head lice, the amount of mature lice found on individuals in the U.S. is relatively small, probably because of our fastidious personal hygiene. A careful search will frequently yield one or two of the crab-like organisms or nits. The identification of eggs less than one-fourth of an inch from the skin indicates active infestation. If the only eggs found are more than that distance from the skin and are empty, it is likely that the disease has already been treated and cured. Crab lice may also be found in the short hairs of the axillae, thighs, and trunk, and occasionally the beard and mustache. In young infants, crab lice may be found in eyebrows and eyelashes.

Prevention and treatment

Until the 19th century, careful body hygiene, frequent clothing changes, and removal of hair from affected areas were the only methods employed in the control of lice. Early in the 20th century a number of treatments including mercuric ointment, heavy metal, crude oil, and kerosene were found to be effective. Although effective, these treatments required several days, were dangerous, and were quite irritating to the skin. Even today, one occasionally sees patients who have treated a louse infestation with kerosene with subsequent development of a florid chemical dermatitis.

The use of DDT, particularly during the epidemics of body lice in World War II, was found to be highly effective. This treatment was especially important because it permitted control of secondary systemic infections, particularly typhus, which was rampant in the Italian theater. Since DDT has been banned, new products, particularly pyrethrins, which are available over the counter, and gamma benzene hexachloride, have come into popular use. Malathion lotion, .05 percent, is not frequently used in the United States.

Treatment of head lice is best accomplished with an appropriate shampoo. The patient should avoid getting the shampoo in the eyes, and the shampoo should not be left in place for longer than the instructions dictate, since it may cause irritation. Some physicians suggest a re-treatment in seven to 10 days to kill lice that have hatched from eggs present at the time of first treatment. Since the success rate of a single treatment is approximately 90 to near 100 percent, this is frequently unnecessary. It is equally effective to simply re-examine the child 10 days after the first treatment for the appearance of new nits close to the skin.

All personal articles should be cleansed at the time of treatment. The eggs and mature lice are killed at hot water temperature (130°F) in 10 minutes, so that laundering in hot water, ironing, or dry cleaning are effective ways of removing the organisms. Since the lice do not persist in the environment for long periods, extensive environmental treatment with insecticides and fogging should be discouraged. Hysteria frequently develops when head lice are diagnosed in schools, so it is important to point out to parents that the mature lice do not survive beyond 48 hours of the weekend, and therefore treatment of the school buildings is unnecessary. If parents are concerned about furniture and carpeting, they should be advised to vacuum these thoroughly. Hairs with attached eggs will be trapped in the vacuum bag, where eggs will die in a period of about one week.

Pubic lice may be similarly treated with an appropriate lotion, as may body lice. One exception is the pubic louse infestation of the eyelashes. Lindane, which is frequently employed in treatment of pubic lice, is quite irritating if it gets into the eyes. A safer treatment is with ophthalmic petrolatum, which will smother the lice. The lice and nits can then be removed with tweezers.

Prevention of spread and isolation

It is important to examine all family members at the time the diagnosis of lice is made and two weeks afterward. All infected persons should be treated. Individuals who share beds with infested individuals should be treated routinely. Other family members need not be. Clothing and bed linen should be sanitized by washing or dry cleaning, and combs and brushes sanitized. Good personal hygiene, daily clothing changes, and not sharing personal items are useful preventive practices.

There is no immunity developed after infestation with lice, so reinfestation can occur, and follow-up examination is needed. It is important to notify the local health department of any diagnosis of lice, particularly in an individual who is part of any regular large group gathering, such as a child from a camp or school or an individual in a community rooming house or a nursing home. Individuals diagnosed as having lice should be placed on wound and skin precautions for 24 hours after adequate treatment. Hospital and nursing-home personnel who develop lice should remain off-duty until they have had adequate treatment for 24 hours.

Bibliography

American Academy of Pediatrics. *Report of the Committee on Infectious Diseases* (17th ed), 1977.

Benenson AS, ed. *Control of Communicable Diseases in Man* (13th ed). Washington DC: American Public Health Association, 1981.

Epstein E, Orkin M, Walsh F. Could that "maddening" itch be lice or mites? *Pat Care* 7: 94, Nov 1, 1973.

Fiumara NJ. The sexually transmissible diseases. *DM* 25(3):1, 1978.

Juranek DD. The nuisance diseases: Pediculosis and scabies. *APIC Newsletter* 4:1, 1976.

Orkin M, Epstein E, Maibach HI. Treatment of today's scabies and pediculosis. *JAMA* 236:1136, 1976.

Parasites Infecting Man. Piscataway NJ: Reed & Carnrick.

11

Tuberculosis

Tuberculosis is a disease of antiquity. Skeletal remains of prehistoric humans indicate the presence of tuberculosis more than 5,000 years ago. During the dark ages and in medieval Europe, the decline in living standards, widespread poverty, oppression, and war led to conditions favoring epidemic tuberculosis. The disease claimed the lives of the famous and unknown equally, causing the death of up to one-fourth of all citizens of some European nations. It was called the white plague because of the waxen, pale countenance of individuals in the terminal stages of pulmonary tuberculosis. The disease was portrayed in art, literature, and music, and many artists themselves suffered from fatal illness. For example, the operas La Boheme and La Traviata depict tuberculosis, and Shelley and Keats both died with extensive pulmonary tuberculosis.

In the contemporary world, the incidence of tuberculosis varies greatly among population groups. In the so-called developed world, the overall incidence of TB is quite low because most of the populations enjoy the benefits of good housing, good sanitation, and adequate nutrition. However, within the developed nations, the population that suffers economic deprivation and hard-core poverty has an incidence of tuberculosis equal to that seen among people dwelling in the developing nations.

Those who work in hospitals contract TB at rates greater than those in Third-World nations today and reminiscent of those of the Middle Ages and the period of the industrial revolution. The acquisition rate of tuberculosis among newly graduated physicians, for example, is approximately one per 100 per year. This is about 10 to 50 times the incidence in the general population of the U.S. Most people involved in health care have a rather generous amount of information concerning the disease. However, because of the episodic presence of individuals with tuberculosis in most hospitals and the sanguine attitude of many physicians concerning the disease, misconceptions about TB are quite common.

Incidence of tuberculosis

Tuberculosis has been declining steadily in the United States throughout the century (Table 11-1). At the turn of the century, the incidence was approximately 500 per 100,000 population. In 1979, the incidence was between 10 and 15 per 100,000. This decline began long before the development of effective chemotherapy for tuberculosis, when treatment was restricted to dietary, climatic, and surgical modalities, which were of

Table 11-1 _____

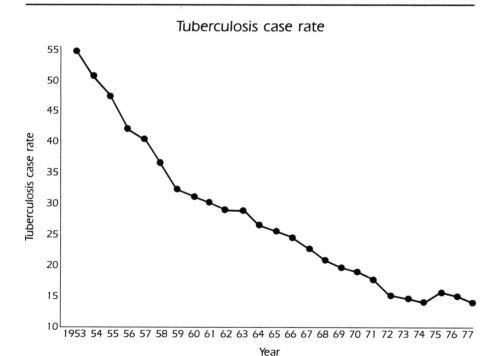

Tuberculosis case rate

Scale at left indicates number of cases per 100,000 population in the United States.

little or no preventive benefit. The decline is largely attributable to improved socioeconomic conditions in the country.

State incidences vary, with Florida, for example, having approximately 20 cases per 100,000 people. And the incidence of TB on Indian reservations and in urban centers with large, crowded, impoverished populations still exceeds 50 per 100,000.

Characteristics of the organism

Mycobacterium tuberculosis is a rod-shaped bacterium approximately 0.3 μ in diameter and 1 to 2 μ in length. When stained, several intrabacterial granules are visible. In its most virulent form, the organism has a capsular, waxy material that causes it to grow in long strands in culture media. This capsular material is referred to as cord factor. *Mycobacterium tuberculosis* requires oxygen for growth, a fact important for understanding the pathogenesis of human TB. It is extremely sensitive to ultraviolet light and dies within a brief period when exposed to sunshine or to the oxidizing materials present in air. These facts have been known for many years and underlie the use of sanitoria with unrestricted air flow, open windows, and much sunlight.

When an individual with tuberculosis organisms present in his sputum coughs, tiny droplets are generated, which harbor only one or two bacilli. The moist protein-bearing sputum surrounding the bacilli desiccates, forming a protective layer that prevents the killing of mycobacteria by sunlight and other oxidizing agents. These dried droplet nuclei remain suspended for prolonged periods because of their static electrical charge. They can then be inhaled into the lungs of other individuals.

Pathogenesis of disease

Droplet nuclei that contain only one to several tubercle bacilli are small enough to pass through the terminal bronchioles into the alveoli. When they do so, they escape the cleansing effect of mucus secreted by the bronchioles and the washing activity of the cilia that line the bronchioles. The tubercle bacilli then may lodge and grow slowly in the alveolus, most often in a lower segment of the lung, the area that receives the most ventilation. Tubercle bacilli divide only once every 14 to 24 hours. As they do, they penetrate the wall lining the alveoli, probably after being ingested but not killed by fixed phagocytic cells in the alveoli, and enter the draining lymphatics. These organisms then float up the lymphatic channel to the lymph nodes lying in the hilus of the lung or the mediastinum, where they are trapped but continue to grow.

Tuberculosis

When the organisms in the lymph nodes overcome the barriers presented by the nonimmune phagocytic cells, they are free to travel into the bloodstream, and spread to other organs, including the kidneys, bone, liver, brain, or the apex of the lung. This hematogenous spread of TB during primary infection probably occurs in almost all individuals who become infected. The area most commonly involved is the lung apex where a high oxygen tension favors growth of the mycobacteria, and they lodge and set up secondary foci.

The symptoms of primary TB are largely those of a mild bronchitis, but can be exaggerated if the host fails to develop a good immune response. In cases of immune failure, multiple nodular tuberculous lesions develop in many organs. These widespread tiny granular lesions, about the size of a millet seed, comprise the condition known as miliary TB. When the disease involves the meninges, meningitis occurs; when the pleura is involved, pleurisy is experienced; if the joints are involved, arthritis; if the lungs are generally involved, the X-rays show the distinctive "snow-storm" of miliary pulmonary TB.

Host response to TB

Most individuals develop an immune response during primary tuberculosis. As the tubercle bacilli grow in various areas of the body, particularly in the lymph nodes, they release materials that adhere to small white blood cells originally derived from the thymus and called thymic or T-lymphocytes. This results in a metabolic burst in the lymphocytes that produces a variety of substances that can help arrest TB. Some of these substances attract phagocytic macrophages to the area of infection. Others immobilize the attracted macrophages, so they cannot exit from the site of infection. Still others stimulate the macrophages to produce more killer substances, which enhances their capability to ingest and kill the tubercle bacilli. In most individuals this immune response is sufficient to immobilize tubercle bacilli and arrest their growth before extensive damage is done. The body then lays down a fibrous capsular wall around the points of initial infection, which may eventually calcify. Calcified foci are found most often in the lower lobe of the lung and the regional draining lymph nodes and are referred to as a Ghon complex.

Tubercle bacilli trapped within these calcified or fibrotic granulomas retain their viability. Under conditions of good host nutrition and health, they are restricted by the defense mechanisms of the host and disease does not occur. However, under circumstances of nutritional deficit, natural disease, or therapeutic intervention in which the body's cellular im-

120

munity is decreased, these trapped organisms are released from controlled growth and may multiply rapidly and overwhelm local resistance. A variety of circumstances are associated with this so-called reactivation, including lymphoma, Hodgkins disease, sarcoidosis, treatment with corticosteroids, X-ray therapy for cancer, acquired immune deficiency, and severe malnutrition.

In reactivation, the multiplying organisms induce an inflammatory response in the host. The inflammatory cells that invade the area of growing tubercle bacilli release substances in an attempt to control bacterial growth. These substances kill the surrounding tissue and convert it to a cheesy mass. This is called caseous necrosis. When this occurs in the lung, the necrosis often spreads to a bronchus. The irritated bronchus causes vigorous coughing, and the walls of the necrotic area may burst. The cheesy material may be coughed out, leaving a hole or cavity in the lung surrounded by the wall of inflammation and advancing tuberculous infection. These cavities are most often in the apices of the lung, where the tubercle bacilli spread during hematogenous primary infection.

As mentioned above, sometimes even the primary phase of TB is not controlled. Under this circumstance, miliary tuberculosis may occur, or the pulmonary infection may progress to involve large segments of the lower portion of the lung, where initial implantation and disease occurred. This so-called primary progressive pulmonary TB has the appearance on X-ray of a bronchopneumonia, but progresses to necrosis and cavitation just as reactivation TB does in the upper lobes.

Most clinical tuberculosis is recognized because of the symptoms associated with reactivation disease. Indeed, it is estimated that more than 90 percent of individuals diagnosed as having active tuberculosis have reactivated dormant tuberculous lesions. Because the reactivation is a slow, indolent process, symptoms are quite few early during reactivation. Only a small, irritating dry cough and minor weight loss are mentioned by most patients. However, as the disease progresses, patients begin to experience progressive weight loss, cough productive of blood-streaked sputum, low-grade fevers rising to 101 to 102°F, heavy perspiration at night with sometimes drenching sweats, hoarseness, easy fatigue, and chest pain.

When the symptoms escape early detection, patients become sources for heavy contamination of the air around them via droplet nuclei. Undetected cases of reactivation TB with cavities and innumerable tubercle bacilli in their sputum are the principal sources of new infections. Identification of all individuals with active or dormant TB is therefore the key to prevention.

Tuberculosis

As in primary tuberculosis, the tubercle bacilli may enter the bloodstream during reactivation disease, with hematogenous spread and the development of secondary lesions elsewhere in the body. These result in presenting symptoms of meningitis, pleurisy, arthritis, osteomyelitis, or even pelvic inflammatory disease. The secondary extrapulmonary lesions established during primary infection, rather than the lung apex, may be the principal source of reactivation, resulting, for example, in bone or renal TB. Individuals whose disease reactivates outside the lung present with fever that eludes an easy explanation. Chest X-rays are frequently normal or reveal only an old Ghon complex. Diagnosis of such extrapulmonary reactivation is a very difficult challenge.

Diagnosis and prevention

Diagnosis of TB takes many forms. Its detection can be as easy as recognition through a classical history or as difficult as biopsy of an adrenal gland or a retroperitoneal lymph node. Chest X-rays, used diagnostically in the past, are no longer the most reliable method. Today the most commonly employed modality for diagnosis of tuberculosis is the skin test, which relies on the principle that when an individual is infected with tubercle bacilli, T-lymphocytes become sensitive to material released from the bacteria. A laboratory preparation of such material, referred to as purified protein derivative, or PPD, can be prepared from the culture medium in which *Mycobacterium tuberculosis* has been grown.

When an appropriate dilution of PPD is injected into the skin of a sensitive individual, sensitized lymphocytes and macrophages migrate into the area with resulting edema and swelling. This local inflammation and swelling, which occurs over a period of 24 to 72 hours, is referred to as a positive skin test. It is thought by most experts that lymphocytes lose their sensitivity to mycobacteria when no live organisms are present in the body. For that reason, a positive test is considered to represent the presence of live active or dormant tubercle bacilli.

It should be recognized that the live mycobacteria contained by host defenses in a Ghon complex are sufficient to maintain a positive skin test. Therefore, positive PPD does not always indicate active disease. Likewise, certain individuals, for reasons imperfectly understood, may have negative skin tests, despite the presence of live organisms within their bodies. This occurs in up to 30 percent of individuals with subsequently diagnosed active tuberculosis.

The most reliable form of skin testing involves the introduction of PPD intradermally by a single needle. This so-called Mantoux test may be done with varying quantities of PPD, which are expressed in unit terminology. These units are arbitrarily related to an equivalent amount of a crude preparation of killed extract of mycobacteria known as old tuberculin. The most dilute form, containing one tuberculin unit equivalent of PPD, is referred to as first strength. Intermediate strength PPD, containing five tuberculin unit equivalents, is the most frequently employed dose.

Individuals strongly suspected of having tuberculosis but having negative skin tests after an intermediate PPD may be subsequently tested with a more concentrated form containing 250 tuberculin unit equivalents. This is called the second-strength PPD. Although more than 95 percent of individuals with tuberculosis have positive skin tests when tested with second-strength PPD, up to one-fourth of all individuals who have positive second-strength PPDs do not have tuberculosis and are therefore referred to as false positive reactors.

An alternative method for large-scale screening of populations is usually referred to as the tine test. A multiple-pronged instrument introduces old tuberculin or PPD through the outer layer of the skin. Although its simplicity facilitates its use for mass screening, in the hands of many individuals the test is neither as sensitive nor as specific as the intradermal Mantoux test. Interpretation of both tests depends on the ability of the tester to recognize the swelling, or induration, of the skin. The swollen area is measured in its greatest dimension. An individual yielding induration of 5 to 9 mm is described as having a questionably positive test. A reaction of 10 mm or more induration is called positive, one of less than 5 mm, negative.

It has recently been recognized that despite the presence of some live tubercle bacilli in certain individuals, circulating T-lymphocytes may lose their sensitivity or react so slowly to PPD as to not give a positive test. This most often occurs in individuals who have had their primary tuberculous infection a number of years previously and have very effectively controlled that infection. Under such circumstances, the first Mantoux test administered may yield a questionable or negative result. However, the small amount of PPD used in the testing is sufficient to remind the T-lymphocytes of their sensitivity—the so-called "booster phenomenon." This stimulated immune memory is manifested by a positive reaction when such individuals are subsequently tested 10 days to two years after the first test. This is an important point to remember in developing plans for large-scale screening of individuals for tuberculin sensitivity.

Since tuberculin sensitivity requires three to six weeks after the primary infection to develop in an individual, one may use the PPD or Mantoux skin test to detect emerging primary infection in individuals exposed to a person with active TB. Since a negative baseline test is necessary to define the emergence of a positive test, contacts of patients with active TB are skin-tested as soon as they are identified. An interval of eight to 10 weeks is permitted to elapse, during which contacts that become infected can develop lymphocyte sensitivity. After this interval, they are skin-tested again. If the test has become positive, they are assumed to have developed primary tuberculosis. If it is still negative, the disease is, for all practical purposes, ruled out. During such screening exercises, certain immune-suppressed states may prevent a positive skin test. Also, certain viral infections from vaccinations of smallpox, measles, and rubella may cause a temporary negative skin test in individuals who indeed have lymphocyte sensitivity to tuberculin.

The simplicity and sensitivity of the Mantoux skin test make it an important vehicle for the detection of TB among individuals with frequent exposure to others with the disease. All hospital employees should have annual skin tests. Those who work in TB hospitals or on pulmonary wards where the incidence of exposure may be quite high should be tested every six months. Individuals who have not had tuberculosis will not develop positive skin tests as a result of repeated testing.

Conversion is defined as development of a positive test (induration of more than 10 mm) in an individual who previously has had a negative (less than 5 mm) or questionable (less than 10 mm) reaction. One year of preventive therapy for converters with the antituberculosis drug isoniazid will reduce the number of surviving bacteria in the individual and will assure that the disease is maximally controlled, or walled-off.

Since approximately one in 10 individuals who have positive skin tests may subsequently develop active tuberculosis, an approach has been developed to reduce this risk of active disease. Under a variety of circumstances, individuals may be given preventive therapy consisting of therapeutic doses of isoniazid daily for one year. With successful completion of a course of preventive therapy, the individual with a positive tuberculin skin test reduces his or her risk of subsequent active TB to that of an individual with a negative skin test, or approximately one in 10,000.

Individuals for whom preventive therapy is recommended include close contacts of those with active pulmonary TB, individuals younger than age 35 who have dormant tuberculosis manifested by a positive TB skin test, any individual who has converted from a negative to a positive skin test over a period of two years or less, and any individual with a positive skin test known to have an underlying disease or condition that increases the risk of reactivation. These diseases and conditions include alcoholism, diabetes, steroid therapy, silicosis, malignancy, sarcoidosis, lymphoma, X-ray therapy, chemotherapy for cancer, and extreme debility in old age.

In addition to the positive skin test, a variety of other studies are useful in the diagnosis of tuberculosis. Not every individual who harbors live mycobacteria has active TB, and the skin test is therefore not diagnostic of active disease. The isolation of *Mycobacterium tuberculosis* from an individual comprises proof of disease. When an actively infected person has a draining lesion, such as a cavity in a lung, an infected focus in a kidney draining into the urine, or even an area of osteomyelitis draining through the skin, tubercle bacilli may be identified in the drainage.

The most rapid method of identification is to stain the organisms and inspect the drainage for their presence. The tubercle bacillus is distinctive in that it retains certain stains more actively than other bacteria. This is taken advantage of in the so-called acid-fast stain, and also in newer techniques employing fluorescent stains. The stain carbolfuchsin, a red stain, is retained by mycobacteria despite vigorous washing with acidified alcohol. These pink-stained bacteria can be relatively easily identified under the microscope. When they are seen, the result is referred to as a positive acid-fast stain. This indicates the presence of mycobacteria, but is not diagnostic of TB since mycobacteria other than *Mycobacterium tuberculosis* are also acid-fast and may be present in clinical specimens without causing disease.

The fluorescent dye rhodamine is likewise actively retained by mycobacteria and causes them to fluoresce. This fluorescence makes the bacteria easily visible under lower magnification than mycobacteria that are stained with carbolfuchsin. The fluorescent staining technique, therefore, has the advantage of permitting the laboratory technician to use a lower power lens and scan larger segments of a smear for the presence of bacteria. The fluorescent stain is at least twice as sensitive for detecting mycobacteria as the classical acid-fast stain.

Specimens for tuberculosis culture, particularly sputum specimens, should be sufficiently large to permit laboratory techniques with a high yield of positives. One of these is the technique of concentrating the specimen by liquefying the sputum and centrifuging the bacteria into a smaller volume. This small volume of concentrated bacteria can be both examined microscopically and cultured.

In the past, standard practice called for the collection of sputum over a 24-hour period to assure an adequate volume, between 5 and 10 ml for concentration. Although an adequate volume was achieved, contaminat-

Tuberculosis

ing bacteria grew so much in these 24-hour sputum specimens that cultures were often overgrown and uninterpretable. For that reason, contemporary practice calls for the collection of a first a.m. sputum specimen. Pulmonary secretions collect in the lung during sleep. When a patient awakens and coughs, large volumes of secretions are produced during the first coughing episode. This first specimen, collected on three consecutive days, is ideal for examination for tubercle bacilli.

The culture is a much more sensitive technique than a smear, since the few mycobacteria collected by concentration are detected when they create colonies on a culture plate. On the other hand, the microscopic detection of tubercle bacilli requires that approximately 10,000 organisms be present per ml of material stained. The culture, however, has the disadvantage of relying upon tubercle bacillus growth. Since the organisms double only every 12 to 24 hours, the creation of colonies sufficiently large to be seen requires three to six weeks. The specificity of culture is better than that of smear. Though nontuberculous mycobacteria are not easily distinguished on a smear and may lead to a false positive, their growth in culture is easily detected by readily available laboratory tests. A positive culture for *M. tuberculosis* is diagnostic of active disease.

Isolation practices

Even before diagnostic procedures are begun, a patient admitted with suspected TB must be handled with special precautions. These are designed to restrict spread of the patient's disease to other patients, employees, and visitors. Since the vehicle for spread of TB is droplet nuclei, only individuals suspected of having pulmonary TB require diligent isolation precautions. Other drainage, although it may rarely be the source of spread, is not nearly so hazardous and can be managed with simple wound and skin precautions. However, when tuberculosis of the lung is suspected, techniques are employed to prevent the patient from coughing out droplet nuclei and others from breathing them in.

Rooms with special ventilation or ultraviolet lights are used to restrict the number of organisms that might be present in the air. Patients are encouraged to wear masks. Individuals entering the room are required to wear masks to prevent their inhaling droplet nuclei from the air. Coughing or sneezing, which is known to expel a great many droplet nuclei, is particularly hazardous. Patients should use tissues to cover mouth and nose when they cough and sneeze and collect in them coughed-up mycobacteria. These trapped organisms no longer present any hazard, and the contaminated tissue can be thrown into a wastebasket.

Necessary care should not in any way be restricted for patients with suspected TB, but unnecessary visiting should be discouraged. Only immediate family and close friends should be allowed visiting privileges. These visitors are important to maintain the patient's psychological balance while he undergoes the rigors of testing for TB. If a patient subsequently has three consecutive negative smears for mycobacteria, he may be removed from isolation, since it has been demonstrated that only those with positive smears cough up enough organisms to be considered a serious threat to others.

If the patient is diagnosed as having pulmonary TB, chemotherapy with two or more drugs should be started within 48 hours. He should be kept in respiratory isolation until two weeks of effective therapy have elapsed. After this period of time, even though organisms may still be present in his sputum, they have been so reduced in virulence by the medication that they are no longer a problem.

Specific therapy for TB is selected based upon the nature of the tubercle bacillus and an estimate of the number of organisms probably harbored by the infected patient. *Mycobacterium tuberculosis* spontaneously develops resistance to any given antituberculous drug about once in every one million bacteria. Therefore, in any individual who is assumed to be infected with more than one million bacteria, more than one drug is employed. Although the lesions of miliary TB contain only as few as 10 and generally no more than 100 bacteria, a tuberculous cavity contains far more than one million organisms. Cavitary TB is the form most frequently treated. Most patients who receive treatment have so-called "bacterial burdens" greater than one million organisms and require multidrug therapy. Such therapy rapidly reduces infectivity, and because of this, many hospitals require that the diagnosis of active disease be followed by prompt initiation of treatment in order to protect employees and other patients.

Although in the hospital a patient being treated for TB requires isolation for two weeks, the patient with active TB whose clinical condition permits a discharge home does not require similar isolation. Close family contacts are assumed to have already been exposed to the patient prior to his admission to the hospital, and others whom he contacts outside the hospital are more likely to be in an outdoors environment and less likely to be immune-compromised and therefore highly susceptible.

Because culture for tubercle bacilli requires three to six weeks, it is not uncommon for the diagnosis to be rendered long after a patient has been discharged from the hospital. This often excites great concern among employees who may have cared for that patient. They can be reassured that the absence of positive smears on such patients, even though they have positive cultures, makes the likelihood of spread of TB extremely small. For that reason, it is not necessary to prepare contact lists and studies of personnel who have cared for a smear-negative but culture-positive patient. On the other hand, if a patient previously hospitalized is discovered to have a positive smear, it is necessary to identify individuals who may have had contact with air contaminated by the patient's secretions in order to detect newly acquired TB.

Obviously, individuals outside the hospital may also have been exposed to a newly discovered tuberculous patient. It is impractical for hospital personnel to attempt to identify all these exposed individuals. Local health departments are charged with this responsibility and generally have adequate personnel. The local health department must be notified of all presumptive or proven cases of pulmonary TB. In addition to screening the patient's family and contacts, many health departments provide free counseling, follow-up, and medication for patients with TB. This is important, since long-term TB therapy requires reassurance, encouragement, and a considerable investment in funds, all of which can be provided through local health agencies.

Older regimens for treatment of tuberculosis require at least two years of medication; however, new agents have been shown to kill the mycobacteria much more rapidly and effectively. Rifampin, one of these new agents, combined with isoniazid is as effective in curing TB in a nine-month course of treatment as older regimens were in two years. Patients must be monitored for side effects of the drugs. With good patient compliance, cure is achieved in at least 99 percent of patients initially treated. Indeed, many authorities equate treatment failure with failure of the patient or physician to follow an adequate regimen. The effectiveness of treatment is judged by a reduction in symptoms, weight gain, improvement in the chest X-ray, disappearance of organisms from the sputum, and, finally, a return to normal good health. Patient education should stress taking medications at the same time every day for the prescribed period. Convincing the patient of the role of medication in curing disease and preventing subsequent reactivation is an essential part of treatment.

Risk of TB in hospital employees

Hospital employees have a considerably greater incidence of development of TB than those in the general population. One to two percent of physicians and other hospital employees acquire the infection each year. If the rate in a particular hospital is in excess of two percent per year, a vigorous prevention program should be instituted and more frequent testing of employees undertaken. For hospital employees, disease acquisition is equated with PPD skin test conversion.

Several studies have now demonstrated that the patient who spreads TB in the hospital is not the one who is recognized as being infected or potentially infected. On the contrary, it is the patient who is not suspected of having the disease and for whom no precautions are taken. Such patients include those suspected of having lung cancer, whose tuberculous lesion mimics a tumor; those suspected of having simple bacterial pneumonia, such as individuals with primary progressive pulmonary TB; and individuals presenting with FUO and a cough.

When any patient has symptoms that may be TB, prompt action should be taken to restrict the spread of the patient's disease and to confirm or rule out its presence. Therefore, three a.m. sputum collections should be ordered as soon as the patient arrives in the hospital. Delay in this procedure simply increases the risk to employees. Five to 10 ml of sputum per sample is sufficient. Certain patients do not produce sputum effectively, often because of the thickness of their secretions. In this case, respiratory therapy may induce sputum with aerosolized saline, or a pulmonary specialist, using fiberoptic bronchoscopy, may obtain secretions by suctioning the lung. To prevent overgrowth of contaminating bacteria invariably present in such specimens, they should be promptly delivered to the laboratory.

In the lab, the specimens are handled under a special bacteriologic hood to avoid unnecessary exposure of the technician and contamination of the specimen. Processing requires several hours, even for a direct-stained smear. If concentration is employed, smears are not available for 24 to 48 hours. Prompt collection of specimens for smear prevents unnecessary prolongation of isolation, with its inconvenience for personnel and the patient, and added expense. Once a patient has had three negative smears, respiratory isolation may be discontinued.

If a patient suspected or known to have active pulmonary TB requires procedures outside the room, or consultation with personnel in the room, the appropriate department should be notified of the diagnosis. If the procedure is elective and can conveniently be delayed, it should be put off until two weeks of chemotherapy have been completed. For essential surgery, special care should be taken in handling anesthesia machines, including the use of disposable circuits and careful cleaning of the machine and the soda lime canister.

In the laboratory, cultures should not be left for three-week intervals, but should be inspected weekly, and any suspicious growth promptly communicated to the unit. Most hospital laboratories lack the facilities for extensive biochemical confirmation and sensitivity testing and send positive cultures to reference or state laboratories for further testing.

Therapy of TB

The drugs employed in the treatment of TB are numerous. They are distinguished by significant differences in toxicity, but all require monitoring. The so-called first-line drugs include isoniazid, rifampin, ethambutol, and streptomycin. Second-line drugs include para-aminosalicylic acid (PAS), capreomycin, ethionamide, pyrazinamide, kanamycin, viomycin, and others. The second-line drugs are significantly more toxic than the first-line drugs.

Isoniazid, the mainstay of treatment of tuberculosis, was first employed clinically in 1952. The customary dose of 300 mg per day achieves, in the usual adult, a sufficient concentration in the blood to inhibit growth of the tubercle bacillus. However, certain individuals, principally Orientals, rapidly metabolize isoniazid in the liver and, therefore, require higher doses. This rapid metabolism of isoniazid is due to genetically determined acetylation of the drug in the liver. This phenomenon of rapid acetylation is rarely seen in Americans because of their extensive interbreeding. With more severe disease or moderately resistant organisms, higher doses may be used, up to a maximum of 700 to 800 mg per day. Certain regimens used with noncompliant patients call for twice-a-week dosing with 1 gram of isoniazid.

The principal toxicity of isoniazid is hepatitis. For this reason, there should be periodic measurements of liver function early in the course of treatment. Some authorities believe if the SGOT rises above twice normal, the drug should be discontinued. An additional side effect is neuritis, frequently manifested by burning in the feet. This is prevented by always giving vitamin B6 with isoniazid. Hypersensitivity and convulsions may also occur. The drug is relatively contraindicated in patients with epilepsy or severe renal disease but can be used, if essential, in modified doses. Finally, isoniazid may cause drowsiness, an effect that can be minimized by dosing at bedtime.

Contemporary treatment of tuberculosis employs rifampin as the second drug in the preferred two-drug regimen. This agent, which is bactericidal for the tubercle bacillus, is given in adults in a usual dosage of 600 mg orally once a day. The drug is toxic to the liver in certain individuals, and this toxicity is increased if patients fail to take the medication every day but treat themselves only intermittently. The drug is excreted in urine, stool, tears, saliva, and even sweat. It appears in these body secretions or excretions in an orange or red color. This may cause concern among patients, and they should be forewarned of it. In addition, rifampin, when excreted in tears, may permanently stain contact lenses. Rifampin interferes with the contraceptive effect of oral estrogens, and women should use other forms of birth control during rifampin treatment.

Ethambutol is the third most commonly used drug for tuberculosis and it, too, is given in combination with isoniazid. The usual dose is 15 mg per kilogram per day. The principal toxic effects are optic neuritis, including loss of visual acuity, color discrimination, and peripheral vision. Individuals on ethambutol should be examined periodically during early stages of treatment to screen for signs of toxicity to the optic nerve.

Streptomycin, the fourth of the so called first-line agents, was developed in the late 1940s, the first effective agent for treating tuberculosis. Its principal disadvantage is that when it is used alone organisms rapidly develop total resistance to the drug. It should, therefore, never be used except in combination with other effective antituberculous drugs. Streptomycin also needs to be given intramuscularly, an added disadvantage. Third, it is notoriously toxic to the eighth cranial nerve, causing deafness in a significant number of individuals who receive more than 14 grams. Since the daily dose is 1 gram, this seriously limits the duration of safe therapy. On the other hand, it is a bactericidal agent for the tubercle bacillus and, therefore, is very effective in combination with other antituberculous agents. Because it is almost exclusively excreted in the urine, streptomycin should be avoided in individuals with renal failure.

The second-line drugs listed above are so classified not because of diminished effectiveness in treating tuberculosis but because of significant toxicity. PAS is toxic to the liver and may cause a significant amount of nausea, vomiting, and gastric burning. Ethionamide and pyrazinamide are also toxic to the liver. Viomycin and kanamycin are toxic to the kidneys and the eighth cranial nerve (hearing and balance). Cycloserine causes psychotic behavior in up to 10 percent of individuals. Thus, use of second-line antituberculous agents requires much closer monitoring of patients than does use of first-line medications.

Nontuberculous mycobacterial infections

In addition to *Mycobacterium tuberculosis,* a wide variety of other mycobacteria, previously called atypical or anonymous mycobacteria, can cause human disease. These organisms may cause lung lesions difficult to distinguish from tuberculosis and equally serious in their long-term consequences. They can cause confusion in the laboratory because they are acid-fast. However, person-to-person transmission of the nontuberculous mycobacteria is not a problem. All of the non-TB mycobacteria together have resulted in only a very few reports of presumed person-to-person transmission. Therefore, isolation is not necessary for such patients. However, since culture identification of a non-TB mycobacterium can require more than a month, such patients are frequently isolated initially in the hospital because they are suspected of having TB. Once the nature of the infecting organisms has been determined, isolation practices are not required.

Infection due to nontuberculous mycobacteria is treated either with antituberculosis drugs or other antibiotics that have been more recently found to be active against these species. Because of frequent problems with resistant mycobacteria, four or more antituberculosis drugs may have to be employed together in treating these infections.

Bibliography

American Lung Association. *Diagnostic Standards and Classification of Tuberculosis and Other Mycobacterial Diseases,* 1974.

Craig CP and Reifsnyder DN, eds. *Infection Control Manual* (4th ed). Tampa: University of Southern Florida, 1978.

Harris HW and McClement JH. Pulmonary tuberculosis. In *Infectious Diseases,* Hoeprich PD, ed. Hagerstown Md: Harper & Row, 1977, pp 318–342.

Lawrence RM. Extrapulmonary tuberculosis. In *Infectious Diseases,* pp 343–349.

Wolinsky E. Nontuberculous mycobacteria and associated diseases. *Am Rev Respir Dis* 119:107, 1979.

12

Aspects of total parenteral nutrition

Prolonged nutritional deficiency is suspected to have serious deleterious effects on the outcome in patients with chronic illness. Surgical and traumatic wound healing, resolution of severe infection, and maintenance of adequate nutrition during prolonged cancer chemotherapy are three conditions that have been favorably influenced by the development of techniques for total parenteral nutrition (TPN). As the list of clinical applications grows, the need for preparing more health providers in prevention, recognition, and management of complications of TPN likewise grows.

The fundamental consideration regarding inclusion of a new indication for supplementary TPN therapy is whether the underlying condition is potentially life-threatening. Because of the complexity and significant complications that surround TPN, its application must be restricted to life-saving circumstances. The second major consideration in prescribing TPN is whether the patient is subject to severe acute or chronic nutritional deficiencies.

Indications for TPN are categorized in three broad groups. The first includes conditions with life-threatening malabsorption of nutrients, such as sprue, Whipple's disease, progressive systemic sclerosis (scleroderma) of the GI tract, and extensive Crohn's disease. Under these circumstances, because the underlying disease may not be reversible, lifelong parenteral alimentation may be required. Techniques for placing semipermanent central venous lines, such as Hickman catheters, to benefit these patients are under active investigation.

In the second category of indications for TPN are patients who are candidates for, or recovering from, surgical correction of gastrointestinal disorders. These include a wide range of diseases with associated gastrointestinal obstruction, including local malignant obstruction with extreme malnutrition, inflammatory obstructions such as diverticular abscess of the ascending colon and high-grade pyloric stenosis due to peptic ulcer disease. Patients who are severely malnourished due to ulcerative colitis are also candidates. Pancreatitis with severe steatorrhea is an indication. Diverticulitis and Crohn's disease are two other inflammatory conditions of the GI tract in which TPN has been employed. Certain congenital GI anomalies, such as Hirschsprung's disease, congenital pyloric stenosis, and atresia of the biliary tract, also are possible indications. In addition, patients with extensive burns who require a great many calories in the acute state and those with chronic wound infections and decubitus ulcers are TPN candidates. Patients with trauma that interferes with alimentation clearly benefit from TPN. Individuals who have had extensive resection of the GI tract and develop resultant severe malabsorption may be maintained for years with TPN.

The third category of indication is medical illnesses that are complicated by malnutrition. This list continues to expand. It now includes severe hypermetabolic states; reversible causes of coma, during which eating is impossible and the placing of a nasogastric tube may promote aspiration; extensive malignant disease for which chemo- or radiation therapy may be employed; reversible acute liver disease, such as acute alcoholic hepatitis and acute viral hepatitis; and various forms of acute and chronic renal failure.

TPN technique

The development of TPN depended upon the discovery of a technique for convenient placement of a central venous line. This was necessary because hyperosmolar solutions given into peripheral veins promptly cause thrombosis. Therefore, the usual hypertonic glucose solutions used in TPN may not be given peripherally. This pattern has been changed recently by the development of lipid emulsions for intravenous use. These can be used as a principal source of calories, a role they fill admirably. Further, they may be conveniently infused in a peripheral vein, since they do not result in acute venous thrombosis.

The technique used to place the IV line used for TPN is very important. TPN is seldom used for short periods. Most patients receive therapy for more than one week. Because the incidence of infectious complications from intravenous catheters rises after the catheters have been in place for four days, careful sterile placement of these lines is a necessity.

The formula used in TPN must be established according to the individual patient's condition. No standard formulation is adequate for all needs. The calorie, trace metal, and supplementary vitamin requirements of children differ markedly from those of adults. Individuals with severe liver or kidney disease may not tolerate heavy loads of nitrogen, thus the amount of amino acids employed in their TPN formulas may need to be restricted. A burn patient metabolizes calories much more rapidly than a patient without burns. A 70-kilogram adult with 60 percent second- and third-degree burns may require more than 5,000 calories a day in order to maintain steady-state nutrition. Under such circumstances, the use of lipid emulsion may reduce the total fluid volume necessary to deliver adequate calories and also reduce the likelihood of complications from chronic hyperglycemia.

A second benefit of lipid emulsion is that for prolonged TPN it largely prevents the development of essential fatty acid deficiencies. For a typical adult, 2,500 to 4,000 ml of solution are generally administered each day, containing up to 5,000 carbohydrate calories, up to 1,000 lipid calories, and up to 150 grams of protein-equivalent amino acids. Electrolytes, including sodium, potassium, magnesium, calcium, and phosphate, are adjusted to maintain normal plasma levels. A variety of vitamins may be given to supplement the available pool. Insulin may be used to control hyperglycemia and its complications.

Complications of TPN

Infection and metabolic derangement are the major complications associated with TPN. Infectious complications are the most common and may be life-threatening. More than 50 percent of infections reported from many centers have been due to fungi. This may be because, unlike bacteria, fungi grow well in a high sugar concentration and tolerate the low pH of some amino acid solutions. In addition, antibacterial ointments are frequently used at the site of venipuncture, which, although they prevent bacterial contamination of the site, permit growth of fungi, particularly *Candida*. The overall rate of blood culture positive septicemia in TPN ranges from less than seven percent in many contemporary studies to more than 30 percent in earlier series of patients. Infections may be introduced directly at the puncture site as a result of contamination of the infusion fluid, or from some remote site as a complication of the underlying host disease, such as burn sites in patients with extensive thermal burns.

Metabolic complications include a variety of nutritional or therapeutic incompatibilities, excess of certain nutrients, and deficiency states. A wide variety of both vitamin deficiencies and toxicities have been reported in patients with chronic TPN. In the era before the development of a safe intravenous lipid emulsion preparation, essential fatty-acid deficiency was common after several months of TPN. Trace metal deficiency is still reported with some frequency, particularly when it is not carefully monitored. Glucose intolerance is a common problem, and frequent checks of blood sugar and CNS function are essential in TPN recipients. Electrolyte and acid base imbalance may occur, either as a result of over-enthusiastic administration of nonphysiologic fluids or because of the diuresis induced by the high glucose load. In such circumstances, the urine produced to carry off the glucose will also carry with it a significant amount of electrolytes, and thus imbalances may ensue. The pharmacist must be alert to incompatibilities of components used in TPN to avoid the complications of precipitation of components, binding of essential components, particularly trace metals, and inactivation of certain medications or components.

Nursing practices to minimize infection complications

The nursing staff has a number of responsibilities in TPN. In some centers, these are assumed by special teams that provide care for TPN for all patients in the hospital. However, in the majority of American hospitals, these responsibilities are still shared among the unit nursing staff. One major responsibility is to assure that solutions are prepared in strictly aseptic environments. Although central preparation of TPN solutions is practiced in some hospitals, many still provide only a base formulation of glucose, amino acids, and lipids to the floor. Other supplements, such as electrolytes and vitamins, are frequently added by unit nurses. Under such circumstances, it is helpful if laminar flow hoods are available on nursing floors. If they are not, traffic in the room where additives are prepared must be halted.

The additives must be mixed aseptically and carefully by individuals who have masks and are wearing sterile gloves. All punctures of TPN-containing vessels should be done aseptically. Once solutions are prepared, they should not be stored for more than 12 hours. Prior to administration, they should be carefully examined for particulate matter and turbidity. Use of a bright light shining through a small hole in a dark room is a superior method for spotting turbidity in solutions, better than the unaided eye. If turbidity or particulate matter are seen, TPN solutions should be returned to the pharmacy.

Another important area of responsibility is the catheter placement. Gowns, masks, and gloves should be used in preparing the setup for placing a central catheter for TPN. Previously, site preparation included defatting the skin with acetone. However, recent studies have concluded that the incidence of heavy bacterial colonization at the puncture site is greater when this practice is used. Therefore, this practice can probably be safely abandoned. It also has the additional hazard of requiring a volatile flammable liquid, the use of which is always of some concern in the hospital environment.

Unless it is impossible to do otherwise, the catheter should not be placed near an active infection or a heavily colonized site, such as the femoral vein. Overgrowth of bacterial flora and vascular invasion can occur rapidly at such sites. The use of an effective antibacterial at the puncture site is essential. Some experts use tincture of iodine followed by alcohol; others employ an iodophor. If the latter is used, it should be left in place for at least four minutes so that adequate iodine is released to provide good asepsis.

After the catheter is placed, iodophor ointment should be used to cover the puncture site. Although this increases the incidence of phlebitis at peripheral sites, this complication has not been reported for central catheters, and the added protection is probably of value. An air-permeable sterile dressing which is transparent at the site may provide prolonged protection. If this is used, it may be practical to cut a small circular opening in the center so that the puncture site itself can have iodophor reapplied periodically. The transparent covering also provides a base to which an occlusive dressing can be applied and removed without irritating the skin, an obvious advantage in prolonged TPN.

Maintenance of the IV catheter is a constant responsibility of the nursing staff. The catheter should be inspected every shift for leakage, and the central vein, most often the subclavian, and surrounding tissue palpated for local tenderness or inflammation. The dressing should not, however, be removed more frequently than every 48 to 72 hours unless there are site complications. When the dressing is removed, strict aseptic no-touch technique should be employed. The site should be carefully cleansed with an iodophor solution and then new iodophor ointment applied with each dressing change.

Total parenteral nutrition

Reducing the risk of infection and complication in patients receiving TPN also requires a number of other measures. Piggyback infusions or other medications should *not* be given through the TPN line. This can lead to incompatibility with precipitation or inactivation of contents, contamination with bacteria or fungi because of the line, or leakage with loss of fluids and subsequent complications. No blood should be drawn from the TPN line, as this probably increases the risk of bacterial infection. An in-line filter of sufficient effectiveness to remove bacteria may be valuable; however, certain of these are incompatible with lipid solutions and there may be leakage of the filter after multivitamin solutions have run through it. Therefore, when the filter is used and if vitamins are to be given, they should be administered with the last unit of solution before the line and filter are to be changed.

The administration tubing connecting the alimentation bottles and the catheter should be changed every 24 hours. If redness, tenderness, or purulent drainage appear at the catheter site, the catheter should be removed and cultured. Some hospitals have found that use of a specially trained TPN team reduces the incidence of sepsis. This is feasible, however, only in larger hospitals or those with a large population requiring this specialized form of therapy.

Diagnosis of sepsis in TPN recipients

As a rule, the occurrence of any fever not present prior to starting parenteral nutrition should suggest catheter-associated sepsis. If a new fever occurs without any other obvious source, the catheter should be removed and the site changed. At the first sign of fever, the nurse should discontinue the infusion and change the fluid and line.

Unlike management of suspected sepsis with routine IVs, a series of cultures are needed to determine the source of infection in TPN. First, fluid should be aseptically collected from the infusion line for culture, either by puncture of the line with a 25-gauge needle after sterile preparation or by capping both ends of the line and sending it intact to the laboratory. This will suffice for determining whether bacterial contamination of the line has occurred. In addition, 10 ml of fluid should be aspirated aseptically from the infusion bottle and sent for culture. The IV site should be inspected; if there is any obvious purulent drainage, this should be cultured, not wiped away and discarded.

If the catheter is to be changed, two blood cultures should be drawn through the catheter. This serves to identify any organisms that may be contaminating the lumen. Next, the skin around the catheter should be carefully cleansed, but only with alcohol. Iodophor should be avoided at this point, since it is difficult to remove and its presence may obscure the subsequent culture results. The catheter should be removed aseptically onto a sterile drape, and the terminal three inches of it clipped with a sterile scissors and rolled over a blood agar plate for semiquantitative culture. This tip of tubing should then be placed in a tube of culture broth. Two other blood cultures should be collected from two different peripheral venous sites in order to determine whether sepsis is occurring. Medical assistance will probably be needed at this time, so that a new central catheter may be placed to continue parenteral alimentation. However, if signs of sepsis occur, these procedures should probably be initiated without delay in order to avoid complications such as shock or remote metastatic infection.

Bibliography

Borgen L. Total parenteral nutrition in adults. *Am J Nurs* 78:224, 1978.

Dudrick SJ. Total intravenous feeding: When nutrition seems impossible. *Drug Ther* 6:11, 1976.

Law DH. Current concepts in nutrition: Total parenteral nutrition. *N Engl J Med* 297:1104, 1977.

Long JM. Practical aspects of parenteral hyperalimentation. *Hosp Phys* 10:35, 1974.

Maki DG, Weise CE, Sarafin HW. A semiquantitative culture method for identifying intravenous-catheter-related infection. *N Engl J Med* 296:1305, 1977.

Montgomerie JL and Edwards JE Jr. Association of infection due to *Candida albicans* with intravenous hyperalimentation. *J Infect Dis* 137:197, 1978.

White PL, Magy ME, Fletcher DC, eds. *Total Parenteral Nutrition.* Acton, Mass: Publishing Sciences, 1974.

Lecture
and Study
Outlines
and Tests

1

The role of the infection control practitioner

Purpose

Hospital employees should be familiar with the expanded role of the infection control practitioner (ICP), the areas of responsibilities it encompasses, the authority it requires, the teamwork necessary to accomplish its goals, and basic principles of infection control.

Learning objectives

- List responsibilities of infection control practitioner.
- Describe "means of transmission."
- Define nosocomial infection.
- Identify the most basic method of preventing spread of infection.
- List infection control resources available in hospital.

Behavioral objectives

- Spot circumstances that foster infection.
- Communicate effectively with the infection control team.

The infection control practitioner

I. Background of infection control.

   A. Original ICPs were "statistics gatherers" hired to fulfill accreditation requirements and prevent litigation due to hospital-acquired infections.

   B. Role was clearly defined—gather data on infections and report them to infection control committee.

   C. Most ICPs were nurses with primary responsibility in other areas or laboratory personnel who had ready access to culture reports and the like.

   D. Infection control has become much more sophisticated in recent years.

      1. ICP now interacts with administration, laboratory, nursing, infection control committee, hospital epidemiologist.

      2. Infection control committee is a base of expertise for developing and evaluating standards of care.

      3. The hospital epidemiologist is a physician with background in infectious diseases and epidemiology.

II. Areas of responsibility of infection control practitioner.

   A. Clinical duties.

      1. Surveillance.

         a.) Collect information regarding patients admitted to hospital with suspected communicable disease, with community- or nursing-home-acquired infections, or who acquire nosocomial infections.

         b.) Compare those who become infected with those who do not, to detect the causes and develop preventive protocols.

         c.) Prepare summary data on patients with infections or communicable diseases.

         d.) Analyze nosocomial infections with help from hospital epidemiologist, infection control committee.

         e.) Report all infections and communicable diseases to local health department.

      2. Employee health (in smaller hospitals, ICP frequently doubles as employee health nurse).

         a.) Review preemployment X-ray, lab and physical exams, and annual laboratory and radiology reports on hospital employees.

         b.) Assist in evaluating employee health problems (colds, flu, rashes, diarrhea).

       c.) Assist in establishing and implementing annual influenza campaigns.

       d.) Develop TB surveillance program for employees.

       e.) Review immunization status of employees.

       f.) Establish health review programs for employees in high-risk areas, such as the dialysis unit.

  B. Administrative duties.

    1. Establish procedures for identifying, monitoring, and eliminating infection hazards in hospital environment, with specific procedures for specific departments.

    2. Be available as resource person for hospital committees.

    3. Attend meetings, participate in committee work relevant to infection control. Helpful committees: audit, policy and procedure, standardization, and head nurse.

  C. Educational duties.

    1. Work with all hospital departments to provide basic orientation in isolation policies and procedures to all new employees.

    2. Establish and update teaching programs for all personnel regarding proper isolation and infection control.

    3. Self-education.

       a.) Review current literature and statutes (local, state, federal) relevant to infectious diseases and infection control.

       b.) Attend workshops and seminars relevant to infectious diseases and infection control.

       c.) Participate in formal courses, especially those offering certification.

          (1.) CDC course in surveillance, prevention, and control of nosocomial infections.

          (2.) College courses in medical microbiology, statistics, and the like.

       d.) Join and participate in professional organizations.

III. Basic principles in infection control.

  A. Chain of infection—source, vector, new host.

  B. Definition of terms.

    1. Infectious agents are bacteria, viruses, fungi, rickettsiae, protozoa.

2. Reservoir—where organisms reside: people, water, soil, equipment.

3. Portal of exit—means by which organisms leave their reservoir: respiratory (coughing and sneezing), intestinal tract (stool), blood (needle puncture or mosquito), skin (shedding or direct contact).

4. Means of transmission—route taken from reservoir to new host: direct and indirect contact, ingestion, airborne (via sneeze), fomites (vehicles), needles, dishes.

5. Portal of entry—means by which organisms enter new host: GI tract, mucous membranes, respiratory tract, broken skin, catheters, IVs.

6. Susceptible host—another person (visitor, patient, staff) with immunosuppression, surgery, burns, diabetes, cardiopulmonary disease.

C. Means for breaking chain of infection.
   1. Good hand-washing technique.
   2. Antibiotic therapy.
   3. Isolation precautions.
   4. Patient placement.
   5. Water purification, careful food storage and preparation.
   6. Patient education.
   7. Sanitation.
   8. Early recognition (diagnosis).
   9. Sterilization/housekeeping.
   10. Product control.

IV. Goal of infection control program—break chain of infection in hospital.
   A. Background on nosocomial infection.
      1. People are more susceptible to infection in hospital than in home, average of five percent develop nosocomial infections (higher rates in teaching and federal hospitals, lower in smaller community hospitals).
      2. Hospital patients are compromised in ability to resist infection.
         a.) Invasive procedures—IVs, Foley catheters, surgery.
         b.) Underlying disease—diabetes, cardiopulmonary disease, and others.

146

      c.) Hospital environment filled with infected patients as sources.

B. Prevent nosocomial infections.

  1. Wash hands thoroughly before and after each patient contact (turn off faucet with paper towel).

  2. Follow isolation procedures—cf. basic five-color system developed by CDC (Figures 1-1 to 1-5, on page 148).

      a.) Yellow sign (Figure 1-1)—strict isolation (rabies, chicken pox).

      b.) Blue sign (Figure 1-2)—protective isolation (oncology, burns).

      c.) Green sign (Figure 1-3)—wound and skin precautions (*Staphylococcus aureus*).

      d.) Brown sign (Figure 1-4)—enteric precautions (hepatitis).

      e.) Red sign (Figure 1-5)—respiratory isolation (tuberculosis).

      f.) Blood precautions.

      g.) Secretion precautions.

  3. Isolate the disease, not the patient.

  4. Resources.

      a.) ICP, epidemiologist, infection control committee.

      b.) Infection control manual, departmental guidelines.

      c.) Health departments, CDC.

Figures 1-1 to 1-5, courtesy of St. Joseph's Hospital, Tampa.

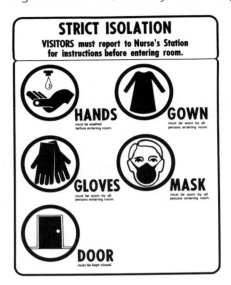

Figure 1-1

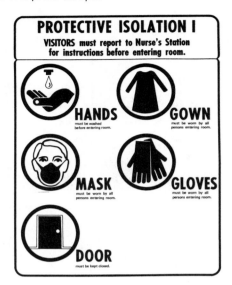

Figure 1-2

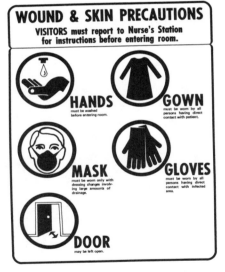

Figure 1-3

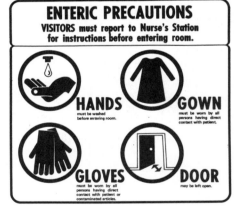

Figure 1-4

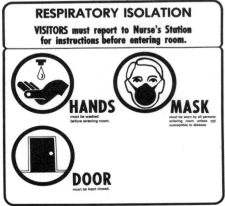

Figure 1-5

T·E·S·T

---

1. Differentiate between direct and indirect contact. Give an example of each.
2. Define nosocomial infection.
3. Match type of isolation with the disease.
   a. strict   _____ *Staphylococcus aureus* wound infection
   b. protective   _____ hepatitis
   c. wound and skin   _____ chicken pox
   d. enteric   _____ tuberculosis
   e. respiratory   _____ leukemia
4. List two infection control resources available in hospitals.
5. What is the most basic method of preventing spread of infection?

Answers are on page 150.

A·N·S·W·E·R·S

1. Direct contact involves immediate physical apposition of an individual to the infected source, such as wound drainage and stool. In indirect contact, a vector transmits infectious organisms from the infected source to the recipient. This vector may be soiled instruments, insects, the air, or the hands of a health-care professional who acquires the organism from an infected source and then deposits it on a susceptible site of another individual.

2. A nosocomial infection is one that was not present or incubating at the time of admission, but occurs during or as an immediate result of hospitalization.

3. c. *Staphylococcus aureus* wound infection
   d. hepatitis
   a. chicken pox
   e. tuberculosis
   b. leukemia

4. The infection control practitioner, the infection control committee, the hospital epidemiologist, the infection control manual, departmental guidelines for infection control.

5. Most authorities consider hand washing to be the most basic method for prevention of infection spread.

2

Gowning, gloving, hand washing, and isolation

Purpose
These procedures prevent spread of communicable disease, reduce unnecessary costs to hospital and patient, and are standard practices of infection control.

Learning objectives
- Identify fundamental routes of spread of communicable disease within the hospital.
- Identify categories of isolation.
- Specify relationships between categories of isolation and routes of disease spread.
- Identify techniques for handling laboratory specimens from isolated patients.
- Select methods necessary for decontamination of articles used in care of infected patients.
- Identify proper principles of isolation technique, including transportation of patient, housekeeping, and rules for visitors.

Gowning, gloving, hand washing, and isolation

Behavioral objectives
- ○ Utilize proper isolation technique.
- ○ Use proper isolation according to disease.
- ○ Communicate information about isolation technique to employees, patients, and visitors.

I. Gowning procedure.
   A. Purpose: A gown is worn to protect visitors and personnel from contamination with secretions and excretions from the patient or his surroundings. The gown should be at least knee length with long sleeves and cuffs and should not be worn outside the isolation area.
   B. Donning procedure.
      1. Before donning gown, wash hands thoroughly.
      2. Slip hands between the back of the gown and shoulders, holding arms high, allowing sleeves to fall over arms.
      3. Tie neck strings.
      4. Tie waist strings securely. Be sure to overlap in back for complete closure.
   C. Removal procedure.
      1. Unfasten waist ties.
      2. Wash hands.
      3. Unfasten neck ties.
      4. Slip hands out of gown, preventing contamination of clothing.
      5. Fold inside of gown over outside.
      6. Roll up so outside portion is inside.
      7. Discard in isolation receptacle.
      8. Wash hands thoroughly.

II. Gloving procedure.
   A. Purpose: Gloves must be worn when indicated. Sterile gloves are used to prevent contamination of patient or increased risk of infection when changing dressings. Nonsterile gloves may be used to prevent contamination of personnel hands in caring for patients with enteric disease or removing contaminated dressings. *Gloves do not replace hand washing.*

Gowning, gloving, hand washing, and isolation

B. Procedure.
1. Gloves are put on after the gown in order that the glove cuffs can be drawn up over the gown sleeves.
2. For sterile gloving.
   a.) Grasp the inside of the cuff of the right glove with the left hand.
   b.) Insert the right hand and pull the glove over the hand.
   c.) This gloved hand can then be inserted under the cuff of the left glove.
   d.) Insert the left hand into the left glove and pull into place, pulling glove cuff over cuff of gown.
   e.) Pull the right cuff well over the wrist.
   f.) The gloves should be removed before the mask and gown and discarded in the isolation receptacle.
   g.) Hands must be washed after gown and gloves are removed.

III. Mask.
   A. Purpose: Principal purpose of wearing a mask is to protect visitors and personnel from airborne infectious droplets.
   B. Procedure.
   1. Wash hands, pick up mask, and adjust over nose and mouth.
   2. Secure ties of mask.
   3. Wash hands, then remove mask by unfastening ties and holding by ties only.
   4. Discard into isolation receptacle.
   5. Masks should not be worn from room to room.

IV. Hand washing.
   A. Purpose: Washing hands between patient contacts is the single most important method to control cross infection.
   B. Procedure.
   1. Stand away from sink to avoid splashing; turn on water to a comfortable temperature.
   2. Wet hands.
   3. Apply soap from dispenser to all surfaces of hands and wrists.

4. Lather hands well, using friction and giving close attention to nails and areas between fingers.

5. Lower hands and rinse off soap under running water, allowing water to flow from above to fingertips.

6. Dry hands using paper towels.

7. Turn faucet off using a dry paper towel.

V. Strict isolation (see Figure 1-1, page 148).

   A. Purpose: For diseases spread by contact, fomites, airborne, and vector routes.

   B. Diseases and duration of isolation.

   1. Anthrax (*Bacillus anthracis*)—for duration of illness.

   2. Burn (major) infected with *Staphylococcus aureus* or Group A *Streptococcus,* or when dressings do not contain the purulent drainage—for duration of illness.

   3. Congenital rubella syndrome—for duration of hospitalization and up to one year for subsequent admissions.

   4. Diphtheriae—until two cultures for *Corynebacterium diphtheriae* are negative after antibiotics have been discontinued.

   5. Herpesvirus (neonatal)—for duration of illness.

   6. Lassa fever—for duration of illness (special facilities recommended).

   7. Marburg virus disease—for duration of illness (special facilities recommended).

   8. Plague (pneumonic)—until culture negative after antibiotics have been discontinued.

   9. *Staphylococcus pneumoniae*—for duration of illness.

   10. *Streptococcus pneumoniae* (not pneumococcus)—for 24 hours after start of effective therapy.

   11. Rabies—for duration of illness.

   12. Skin infection (major)—for duration of illness.

   13. Smallpox—until all crusts are shed.

   14. Vaccinia (generalized)—for duration of illness.

   15. Varicella (chicken pox)—for seven days after first crop of vesicles appear. Any asymptomatic susceptible patient who has been exposed and who must be hospitalized should be isolated for three weeks after the exposure. This category also includes disseminated zoster (shingles).

C. Procedural points.
   1. Room—private room mandatory; negative pressure suggested.
   2. Gown required for all who enter.
   3. Masks must be worn by all who enter room.
   4. Hand washing required before entering and on leaving.
   5. Sphygmomanometer and stethoscope must remain in room. On terminal cleaning, double-bagged and labeled "Strict Isolation." Sent for decontamination.
   6. Needles and syringes—placed in puncture-proof container in patient's room. Sealed for steam autoclaving or incineration.
   7. Dressings and tissues—double-bagged, labeled, incinerated.
   8. Urine and feces—disposed of into sewer system.
   9. Linen—removed carefully, double-bagged, and labeled "Isolation."
   10. Dishes.
       a.) Disposable dishes and items—placed in wastebasket.
       b.) Leftover food—wrapped and discarded in wastebasket or flushed down toilet.
       c.) Liquids—poured in sink drain or toilet.
       d.) Reusable dishes, trays, and utensils—double-bagged in impervious bags clearly marked "Isolation" and sent for decontamination. Personnel must wear gloves when handling contaminated articles and wash hands before handling clean dishes.
   11. Clothing.
       a.) Laundered or sterilized.
       b.) Washed at home according to specific instructions.
   12. Laboratory specimens.
       a.) Lid securely closed on all specimen cups.
       b.) Placed in transparent double bag with lab request on outside bag.
       c.) Bag properly labeled "Contaminated" or "Strict Isolation."
   13. Books, money, letters, toys: No special precautions unless contaminated with patient's secretions, and those should be disinfected or destroyed.

Gowning, gloving, hand washing, and isolation

14. Charts.
    a.) Kept outside of patient room.
    b.) Disposable writing equipment available in room.
15. Visitors.
    a.) Immediate family only.
    b.) One visitor at a time.
    c.) Visitors instructed in proper donning of protective clothing.
16. Transporting patients.
    a.) Service notified of patient's highly communicable disease.
    b.) Patient wears a full-length clean isolation gown.
        (1.) Clean cotton blanket lining wheelchair and surrounding patient.
        (2.) Clean cotton blanket covering patient on a cart, leaving face exposed.
    c.) Patient wears a high-efficiency disposable mask.
    d.) Strict isolation card accompanies patient.
17. Concurrent cleaning.
    a.) Protective clothing worn.
    b.) Wiping cloths discarded in a receptacle in room.
    c.) Cleaning equipment disinfected in room.
    d.) Mop heads double-bagged and then laundered and dried.
    e.) Dirty water discarded and bucket disinfected in room.
18. Terminal disinfection.
    a.) Protective clothing for housekeeping personnel.
    b.) Air filters changed from air conditioner.
    c.) Airing period of one to two hours with window open and door closed prior to terminal cleaning may be indicated.
    d.) All contaminated receptacles emptied and rinsed, double-bagged, and sent for sterilization. Separate small articles can be steam- or gas-autoclaved.
    e.) All contaminated trays should be double-bagged and sent for sterilization.

Gowning, gloving, hand washing, and isolation

VI. Protective isolation (see Figure 1-2, page 148).
   A. Purpose: to prevent contact between potentially pathogenic organisms and infected persons who have seriously impaired resistance.
   B. Diseases.
      1. Uninfected burns.
      2. Congenital or acquired severe immune deficiency (except for AIDS, blood precautions).
      3. Immunosuppressive radiation or chemotherapy.
      4. Lymphomas and leukemia.
      5. Severe dermatitis.
   C. Procedural points.
      1. Private room necessary with trash and linen containers kept outside patient's room.
      2. Gowns and masks necessary for all persons entering the room.
      3. Hand washing necessary before entering and on leaving the room.
      4. Gloves worn for direct patient contact.
      5. Material and equipment decontaminated before taken into the room and left in the room, if at all possible.
      6. Transporting the patient curtailed.
      7. Used linens not considered contaminated; some patients, such as burn patients, may require sterile linen.
      8. Visitors limited and instructed in the use of protective clothing.
      9. Cleaning routine, but with housekeeping personnel in protective clothing.
      10. Dishes and specimens—no special precautions.

VII. Respiratory isolation (see Figure 1-5, page 148).
   A. Purpose: To prevent transmission of organisms by droplets or droplet nuclei that are coughed, sneezed, or breathed into the environment.
   B. Diseases and duration of isolation.
      1. Measles—for four days after onset of rash.
      2. Meningococcal meningitis—for 24 hours after start of effective therapy.

      3. Meningococcemia—for 24 hours after start of effective therapy.

      4. Mumps.

      5. Pertussis (whooping cough).

         a.) No therapy—for three weeks after onset of cough paroxysms.

         b.) With therapy—for seven days after therapy.

      6. Rubella—for five days after onset of rash.

      7. Tuberculosis—for two weeks after adequate therapy.

C. Procedural points.

      1. Private room with air control for tuberculosis; tuberculosis patient may share room with another already on therapy.

      2. Gowns not necessary.

      3. Masks worn by susceptible personnel and visitors who remain in the room for a prolonged period. Patients considered to be high transmitters, such as those with untreated tracheal or laryngeal tuberculosis, might need to wear masks while personnel or visitors are in the room.

      4. Hand washing necessary.

      5. Gloves not necessary.

      6. No special precautions for the following.

         a.) Sphygmomanometer and stethoscope.

         b.) Needles and syringes.

         c.) Urine and feces.

         d.) Dishes.

         e.) Linen.

         f.) Books, magazines.

         g.) Thermometer.

         h.) Clothing and personal effects.

         i.) Patient's chart.

      7. Visitors.

         a.) Immediate family only.

         b.) Two visitors at a time.

         c.) Those who must wear masks instructed by nursing service.

8. Patients being transported are to wear high-efficiency masks, except those who agree to cover nose and mouth when coughing.

9. Cleaning personnel alerted to potential hazards and instructed as to proper precautions, including the use of the mask when indicated. Trash containing tissues patient used when coughing should be double-bagged.

10. Terminal disinfection of well-ventilated room can be done as soon as patient leaves. Windows open and doors closed for a period of one to two hours may be necessary prior to terminal cleaning.

11. Respiratory therapy equipment wrapped and returned to central supply or respiratory therapy department, or for reprocessing.

12. Laboratory specimens—no special handling, but labeled "Tuberculosis."

VIII. Enteric precautions (see Figure 1-4, page 148).

    A. Purpose: To prevent direct or indirect contact with infected feces or heavily contaminated articles. Transmission of infection depends on ingestion of pathogen.

    B. Diseases and duration of precautions.

        1. Cholera—for duration of illness.

        2. Diarrhea with suspected infectious etiology—for duration of illness or until infectious etiology is disproved.

        3. Enterocolitis—until there is one negative culture after antibiotics have been discontinued.

        4. Gastroenteritis—for duration of illness.

            a.) Enteropathogenic *E. coli*.

            b.) Enterotoxigenic *E. coli*.

            c.) *Salmonella* species.

            d.) *Shigella*.

            e.) Pseudomembranous colitis.

            f.) *Yersinia enterocolitica*.

            g.) *Campylobacter jejuni*.

        5. Typhoid—for duration of stool carriage.

    C. Procedural points.

        1. Room.

            a.) Separate room for children.

b.) Adults in multipatient rooms, unless they have fecal incontinence or behavioral problems. Incontinent patients should not share toilet facilities.

2. Gowns for direct contact with patient or his excretion.
3. Proper hand washing required.
4. Gloves for direct contact with potentially contaminated articles, such as urinals, bedpans, commodes, linens.
5. Needles and syringes placed in an impervious puncture-resistant container, double-bagged, and incinerated or steam-autoclaved. Disposables should be used with hepatitis patients.
6. Dressings placed in impervious sealed plastic bag, discarded in wastebasket, and incinerated without being opened.
7. Urine and feces flushed down the toilet. If patients share bathroom, each patient must wash hands before and after using toilet facilities.
8. Utensils wrapped in impervious bag marked appropriately for isolation and sent for decontamination and sterilization.
9. Linen.
   a.) Used linen placed in bag in room or close to patient's bed.
   b.) Water-soluble bags should be placed unopened in washing machine. Regular laundry bags should not be sorted, but placed directly into washing machine.
   c.) Mattress and pillows covered with impervious plastic should be cleaned with germicidal detergent.
10. Food.
    a.) Leftover food wrapped and discarded in wastebasket or flushed down toilet.
    b.) Liquids poured down sink or toilet.
11. Dishes.
    a.) Disposables placed in wastebasket.
    b.) Nondisposables placed in clean impervious plastic bag and sent to kitchen on regular cart.
    c.) Personnel should wash hands after handling contaminated articles.

12. Clothing laundered or sterilized before being sent home. Otherwise, placed in double bags with home laundering instructions.

13. Laboratory specimens.
    a.) Specimens placed in sterile labeled containers with secure lids.
    b.) Double-bag container in clear plastic bag labeled appropriately for isolation. Laboratory request placed on outside of bag.
    c.) Blood specimens for hepatitis cases labeled "Blood Precautions."

14. Contaminated articles wiped clean with germicide detergent solution.

15. Chart—no special precaution.

16. Visitors limited and instructed on proper isolation technique.

17. Clean sheets and pajamas used in transporting patients.

18. Cleaning personnel instructed about potential hazards, with careful attention to proper precautions to be used while cleaning room.

19. Terminal disinfection.
    a.) Urinals and bedpans placed in an impervious plastic bag labeled "Isolation" and sent for decontamination and sterilization.
    b.) Disposable items placed in wastebasket lined with impervious plastic bag. On removal, liner is closed securely and contents incinerated.

20. Removable and easily handled parts of special instruments placed in impervious bag and sent to be decontaminated and sterilized. Other parts are wiped off with germicidal solution and sent for decontamination.

21. Procedure trays sent for decontamination after separating disposables, autoclavables, and linens into different bags.

IX. Wound and skin precautions (see Figure 1-3, page 148).
   A. Purpose: To prevent direct contact with infected wounds and heavily contaminated articles.
   B. Diseases—isolate until drainage ceases or is completely contained in dressings.

Gowning, gloving, hand washing, and isolation

1. Wound and skin infections, covered or uncovered. (Patients with extensive burn infections or infections due to *Staphylococcus aureus* or Group A *Streptococcus* with copious drainage should have strict isolation.)
2. Herpes zoster, localized (shingles).
3. Gas gangrene/*Clostridium perfringens.*
4. Impetigo.
5. Plague, bubonic.
6. Endometritis.
7. Highly resistant epidemic strains of any species may require special precautions (cohorting or strict isolation).

C. Procedural points.
   1. Private room or proper patient placement; may place with nonsurgical, non-high-risk patients.
   2. Gowns for persons having direct patient contact to prevent contaminating uniforms.
   3. Masks not necessary, except during dressing change with copious drainage.
   4. Gloves for persons having direct contact with the infected area or contaminated articles. Two sets of gloves must be used when dressings are changed—the first set when removing the dressing and another set when applying new dressings; wash hands between glovings.
   5. Hands washed on entering and leaving the area and when otherwise indicated.
   6. Dressings double-bagged for disposal.
   7. Linens double-bagged.
   8. Visitors to have no contact with infected area or wound.
   9. Infected areas covered during transport. Soiled areas on transport vehicle to be cleansed with disinfectant.
   10. Routine cleaning done with proper precautions for linen, dressings, and trash.
   11. Instruments labeled "Contaminated" or "Isolation" and sent to be decontaminated.
   12. Special procedure trays need no special precaution unless they are contaminated with drainage. Double-bag these for special decontamination.
   13. Lab specimens require no special handling, except for labeling "Wound and Skin Precautions."

Gowning, gloving, hand washing, and isolation

X. Secretion precautions (Figure 2-1, page 165).
  A. Purpose: To prevent spread of disease by secretions coming in contact with open wounds or mucous membranes of the recipient.
  B. Diseases and duration of precautions.
    1. The following should have secretion precautions for lesion drainage.
        a.) Actinomycosis, draining—for duration of drainage.
        b.) Anthrax, cutaneous—until cultures are negative.
        c.) Brucellosis, draining—for duration of drainage.
        d.) Burn infection, dermatitis, and minor wound infections—for duration of drainage.
        e.) Candidiasis, mucocutaneous—for duration of illness.
        f.) Coccidioidomycosis, draining—for duration of drainage.
        g.) Conjunctivitis, bacterial—for 24 hours of effective therapy.
        h.) Conjunctivitis, viral—for duration of illness.
        i.) Gonorrhea—for 24 hours of effective therapy.
        j.) Granuloma inguinale—for duration of illness.
        k.) Herpesvirus hominis, localized—for duration of illness.
        l.) Keratoconjunctivitis, infectious—for duration of illness.
        m.) Listeriosis—for duration of illness.
        n.) Lymphogranuloma venereum—for duration of illness.
        o.) Nocardiosis, draining—for duration of illness.
        p.) Orf—for duration of illness.
        q.) Syphilis, cutaneous or mucous membrane—for 24 hours of effective therapy.
        r.) Trachoma, acute—for duration of illness.
        s.) Tuberculosis, extrapulmonary draining—for duration of drainage.
        t.) Tularemia, draining—for duration of drainage.
    2. The following should have secretion precautions for oral transmission.
        a.) Herpangina—for duration of hospitalization.
        b.) Herpesvirus hominis, oral—for duration of illness.
        c.) Infectious mononucleosis—for duration of illness.

d.) Melioidosis, pulmonary—for duration of illness.
e.) Mycoplasma pneumonia—for duration of illness.
f.) Pneumonia, bacterial, not covered elsewhere—for duration of illness.
g.) Psittacosis—for duration of illness.
h.) Q fever—for duration of illness.
i.) Respiratory infection, acute, not covered elsewhere—for duration of illness.
j.) Scarlet fever—for 24 hours of effective therapy.
k.) Streptococcal pharyngitis—for 24 hours of effective therapy.

C. Procedural points.
1. Private room, gown, mask not necessary.
2. Gloves required for all contact with contaminated secretions.
3. Hand washing required before entering and on leaving the room.
4. Instruments, needles, and syringes need no special precautions.
5. Dressings and tissues double-bagged, labeled, and incinerated.
6. Urine and feces need no special precautions.
7. Linen double-bagged only if grossly contaminated with secretions.
8. Dishes need no special precautions.
9. Clothing needs no special precautions.
10. Laboratory specimens need no special precautions except to be labeled with suspected diagnosis.
11. Charts need no special precautions.
12. Visitors follow prescribed precautions.
13. In transporting patients, receiving service to be notified of suspected disease. Any wound should have a clean dressing. Transportation vehicle should be covered with a clean sheet.
14. Concurrent cleaning done with usual practices.
15. Terminal disinfection done with usual practices.

Gowning, gloving, hand washing, and isolation

Figures 2-1 and 2-2, courtesy of St. Joseph's Hospital, Tampa.

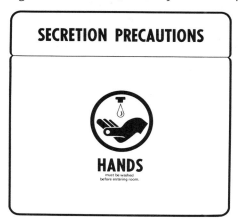

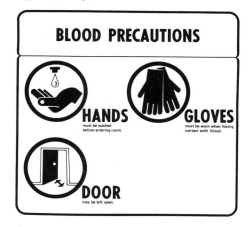

Figure 2-1   Figure 2-2

XI. Blood precautions (Figure 2-2).
   A. Purpose: Arthropod-borne diseases, such as encephalitis or malaria and viral hepatitis, are almost exclusively transmitted in the hospital environment by blood or blood products. Thus, special precautions should be taken in handling blood of such individuals.
   B. Diseases and duration of precautions.
      1. Arthropod-borne viral diseases—for duration of hospitalization.
      2. Hepatitis, viral, type A, B, or non-A, non-B—for duration of hospitalization.
      3. Malaria—for duration of hospitalization.
      4. Acquired immune deficiency syndrome (AIDS)—duration of hospitalization.
   C. Procedural points.
      1. Private room, gowns, and masks unnecessary, except that incontinent individuals with hepatitis A require private toilet facilities and gowns. Gowns recommended for AIDS.
      2. Hand washing necessary before entering and on leaving the room.
      3. Gloves worn whenever there is likelihood of blood contamination of hands and when handling excreta.

4. Articles and equipment require no special care unless contaminated with blood or excreta.
5. Patient may be transported on a clean sheet. Receiving department should be notified of communicable illness.
6. Linens not considered contaminated unless blood-soiled.
7. No special limitations for visitors.
8. Routine concurrent cleaning.
9. Specimens labeled "Blood Precautions"; no special precautions for dishes.
10. Routine terminal cleaning.

T·E·S·T

1. Identify five categories of isolation.
2. Explain why isolation techniques vary with diseases.
3. What is the best way for personnel to prevent spread of infections in the hospital?
4. What is the purpose of wearing protective clothing (gown and mask)?
5. When should sterile gloves be worn?
6. When should unsterile (clean) gloves be worn?

A·N·S·W·E·R·S

1. Strict, protective, respiratory, enteric, wound and skin, secretion, and blood precautions are categories of isolation.

2. Isolation techniques are designed to restrict spread of infections, not to isolate patients. Because not all diseases are spread by the same methods, they may be segregated into categories of isolation, thus permitting greater freedom of movement for patients and more efficient patient care.

3. Personnel should understand and use the infection control policies of the hospital. Foremost among these are appropriate care and management of infected patients and careful, frequent hand washing.

4. Protective clothing prevents contamination of one's own clothing, which might serve as a vector for transmission of infection. A mask protects the wearer from inhalation of organism-bearing particles.

5. Sterile gloves are worn to prevent introducing new pathogens into open wounds or normally sterile body areas. For example, sterile gloves should be used by personnel changing dressings on surgical wounds and suctioning patients with endotracheal tubes.

6. Unsterile (clean) gloves are worn to protect the hands of the wearer from contamination. For example, unsterile gloves should be worn by personnel removing dressings from patients with infected wounds, removing a Foley catheter, or handling excreta from patients with enteric infections.

3

Patient placement

Purpose

Patient placement guidelines are established so that patients with compromised natural resistance to infection (high-risk patients) and clean surgical patients are not assigned to rooms with patients with communicable infections or potential infections. All patients should be identified on admission according to diagnosis, current surgical procedure, and any underlying medical condition.

Learning objectives

○ Understand rationale for patient placement.
○ Identify the classifications for patient placement.
○ State definition for high-risk patient.
○ Define surgical categories of patients.
○ List exceptions to placement.

Behavioral objectives

○ Classify patients on admission according to diagnosis.
○ Choose appropriate room assignments.
○ Protect high-risk and clean surgical patients from communicable nosocomial infections.
○ Evaluate patient placement on a nursing unit.

Patient placement

I. Method
  A. Patients identified on admission according to several criteria.
    1. Diagnosis.
    2. Planned surgical procedure.
    3. Underlying medical condition.
  B. Coordinated effort and close communications.
    1. Staff nurse does medical evaluation and classification.
    2. Physician provides additional information on health status. Physician has legal responsibility for patient placement.
    3. Admitting personnel control bed assignments. They know of bed needs for incoming patients and status of patients already admitted.
    4. ICU, one-day surgery, and emergency department nurses frequently have high-risk or infected patients who need bed reassignment.
    5. Nurse epidemiologist arbitrates problems in placement, educates, reviews, corrects deficiencies.
  C. Daily assessment of patient's status.
  D. Classification system.
    1. High-risk patient (susceptible).
      a.) Definition: Patient who has greater-than-normal susceptibility to infection.
      b.) Examples: Cancer, advanced leukemia of any type, lymphomas, treatment with anticancer or leukemia drugs, Hodgkins disease, lupus erythematosus, pregnancy, sickle-cell anemia, agranulocytosis, kidney transplant, burn patient with extensive dermatitis, steroid therapy.
      c.) May be placed with patients who are not infected or likely to become infected.
      d.) Roommate for high-risk patients.
        (1.) Any other uninfected medical or other high-risk patient.
        (2.) Surgical patient in the clean or clean-contaminated categories.
        (3.) No "suspect patient" or any patient having an infection or contagious disease.
        (4.) Special circumstance—catheterized patient without UTI should not be placed with catheterized patient with UTI.

2. Suspect patient (spreader).

   a.) Definition: Patient who because of infection or incontinence can spread infectious microorganism to other patients.

   b.) Examples: Bedsores, draining; chronic lung disease; conjunctivitis, draining; cysts, draining; diarrhea, if possibly contagious; febrile patient (FUO) suspected of having underlying infection, unless the physician documents that the patient is not contagious; pneumonia; bronchitis; severe URI; Foley and UTI.

   c.) May be placed with any patient who would not fall in the high-risk or clean or clean-contaminated surgical categories.

3. Infected patient.

   a.) Definition: Patient with a contagious disease (either confirmed or suspected) or with any wound that is draining purulent material.

   b.) Placement depends on isolation or precautions required.

      (1.) Patient in this category must not be placed with high-risk or clean or clean-contaminated surgical patient.

      (2.) Patients on strict or respiratory isolation must be in private rooms—if possible, with separate negative pressure air exchange and anteroom.

4. Medical patient.

   a.) Definition: Nonsurgical patient who is not included in any other category.

   b.) Examples: Acute MI, CHF, pulmonary embolus, GI bleeder.

   c.) May be placed with any patient in any category, unless prohibited by isolation or precaution.

E. Classification and placement of surgical patients.

1. Clean surgery.

   a.) Definition: A clean wound is a nontraumatic uninfected operative wound in which the respiratory, alimentary, and oropharyngeal tracts are not entered. Clean wounds are elective, primarily closed, and undrained wounds.

   b.) Examples: Eye surgery, cardiac surgery, neurosurgery, mastectomy, elective C-section, orthopedic (reconstructive) surgery, vascular surgery, thyroid and parathyroid surgery.

c.) Placement.

(1.) May be placed with other clean surgical patients, high-risk patients, or noninfected medical patients.

(2.) May be placed with selected clean-contaminated surgical patients if necessary.

2. Clean-contaminated surgery.

a.) Definition: Clean-contaminated wounds are operative wounds in which the respiratory, alimentary, or genitourinary tract is entered without unusual contamination or wounds that are mechanically drained.

b.) Examples: Appendectomy (elective); biliary tract entered in absence of infected bile; dental surgery; gastrectomy; hysterectomy; hemorrhoidectomy; therapeutic abortion; pilonidal cystectomy; nose and throat surgery; vaginal delivery (with membranes ruptured within 24 hours); genitourinary tract entered in absence of infected urine; GI or respiratory tract surgery without significant spillage; D&C without infection.

c.) May be placed with any other patient in this category, a high-risk patient, noninfected medical patient, or clean surgical patient.

3. Contaminated surgery.

a.) Definition: Contaminated wounds include open fresh traumatic wounds; operations in which a major break in sterile technique occurred; large bowel resection with spillage; and incisions encountering acute nonpurulent inflammation.

b.) Examples: Fresh colostomy and closure of colostomy; compound fracture less than 24 hours old; gunshot wound; acute cholecystitis, acute appendicitis (appendectomy); rectal surgery.

c.) Patients in this category may be placed together or may be placed with nonsurgical patients who are not high-risk. They should not be placed with surgical patients in other categories.

4. Dirty and/or infected surgery.

a.) Definition: Surgery on old traumatic wounds or on patients with clinical infection, perforated viscera, or on wound and skin precautions. The definition of this category suggests that the organisms causing postop infection are present in the operative field before surgery.

b.) Examples: Perforated viscus; traumatic wound more than 24 hours old or with retained devitalized tissue or foreign body.

c.) May be placed with others in this category or with medical patients who are not high-risk.

II. Exceptions.

A. When proper placement is not possible at the time the patient is admitted, correct accommodations should be made as soon as possible. Document need for all exceptions in writing.

B. Necessary care should not be denied simply because of problems in patient placement.

T·E·S·T

1. List the four categories by infection status of surgical wounds.
2. True or False. A patient with Foley catheter and *E. coli* urinary tract infection may safely share a room with an uninfected Foley-catheterized patient.
3. Which of the following are responsible for patient placement?
   a. admitting physician. b. admitting office.
   c. admitting nurse.   d. infection control practitioner.
   e. all of the above.
4. Match the patient with the placement category:
   a. high-risk   ＿＿＿ leukemia, acute
   b. spreader   ＿＿＿ total hip replacement
   c. medical   ＿＿＿ staphylococcus wound infection, draining
   d. clean surgery   ＿＿＿ acute myocardial infarction
                         ＿＿＿ shingles
                         ＿＿＿ inguinal herniorrhaphy

Answers are on page 174.

Patient placement

A·N·S·W·E·R·S
---

1. Clean, clean-contaminated, contaminated, and dirty are categories of surgical wounds in terms of infection status.
2. False.
3. e. All those mentioned in a–d.
4. a. leukemia, acute
   a. total hip replacement
   b. staphylococcus wound infection, draining
   c. acute myocardial infarction
   b. shingles
   d. inguinal herniorrhaphy

4

Urinary tract infection

Purpose

This section reviews the urinary system, the signs that indicate the presence of infection, the symptoms of infection, proper methods of specimen collection, and the steps to take to prevent urinary tract infection.

Learning objectives

○ Know the characteristics of urine that indicate infection.

○ Know the incidence of urinary tract infection and related septicemia in the hospitalized patient.

○ List the signs and symptoms of urinary tract infection.

○ Delineate the common approaches to treatment and prevention of urinary tract infection.

Behavioral objectives

○ Recognize urinary tract infection by its signs and symptoms, including the characteristics of infected urine.

○ Collect a urine specimen for culture.

○ Take proper steps in care of the Foley catheter and closed drainage system to prevent urinary tract infection.

○ Care for the patient on intermittent catheterization or the patient with a leg bag by following the basic steps of asepsis.

Urinary tract infection

I. Statistics.
  A. Approximately 40 percent of all hospital-acquired infections are of the urinary tract (UTI).
  B. Straight catheterizations have one percent to five percent infection rate.
  C. Foley catheterizations are a major cause of UTI.
    1. More than 400,000 patients a year develop catheter-associated UTIs.
    2. Ninety to 95 percent of patients with Foley catheters become infected within four days if the system is an open system; 30 percent or less if the system is closed.
  D. Nearly 75 percent of patients with hospital-acquired UTIs have had some form of urologic instrumentation.
  E. UTIs are a cause of gram-negative sepsis.
    1. One percent develop sepsis.
    2. There is a 30 to 50 percent mortality rate in sepsis, causing 50,000 deaths a year in the U.S.

II. Normal urine vs. infected urine.
  A. Appearance.
    1. Clear amber is normal.
    2. Cloudiness in a freshly voided specimen may indicate the presence of blood, pus, bacteria, or crystals or any combination of these.
  B. Odor.
    1. Aromatic, not unpleasant.
    2. Ammonia odor may indicate infection, particularly *Proteus* species, which splits urea into CO_2 and ammonia.
  C. Microscopic examination of urine.
    1. Red blood cells.
      a.) An occasional cell is considered normal.
      b.) Many cells are a sign of infection, tumor, trauma, or glomerulonephritis.
    2. White blood cells.
      a.) Greater than 10 or clumps of WBCs in a noncentrifuged specimen are significant and indicate a suppurative process.
      b.) White cell casts are shed from infected tubules in pyelonephritis.

3. Bacteria.

    a.) None are seen in normal unspun urine.

    b.) Improperly collected urine from women may contain many bacteria from the perineum.

    c.) Infected urine shows bacteria microscopically.

D. Concentration and output.

    1. After an overnight fast, specific gravity is generally 1.025 or higher; in pyelonephritis, generally less than 1.015.

    2. Normal adult output is 1,500 cc per day.

E. Sites and pathogenesis of UTI.

    1. Most UTIs arise from bacteria ascending the urethra. Distal $\frac{1}{2}$ cm of female and 1 to 2 cm of male urethra are normally colonized with bacteria.

    2. Due to short urethra, among other likely causes, women have more UTIs than men (2.5 to 10 percent per year for women; 0.1 percent per year for men).

    3. Bacteria in bladder may be eliminated by urination or inhibited by organic acids and low pH in urine.

    4. If bladder is successfully infected (cystitis), bacteria may enter ureters. Endotoxin from gram-negative bacteria can paralyze ureteral peristalsis, permitting bacteria to swim up to and infect kidney (pyelonephritis).

    5. Infections in kidney may spread to perirenal space (perinephric abscess); in male, bladder may infect prostate (prostatitis).

    6. Occasionally, bacteria from blood (septicemia) infect kidney hematogenously (pyelonephritis).

III. The urine culture.

A. The clean-catch urine specimen.

    1. Use a sterile container.

    2. Instruct the male patient in cleansing of the meatus, female patient in holding labia apart during and after cleansing.

    3. Make sure patient voids a small amount prior to collecting specimen.

    4. For women, two consecutive morning specimens are necessary for accurate testing. There must be 100,000 of same organism in each specimen to indicate infection.

       5. Specimen must go immediately to the lab to prevent overgrowth of organisms.

  B. The catheterized patient.

     1. The straight catheter.

       a.) Use a sterile container and sterile technique.

       b.) Take specimen immediately to the laboratory.

     2. The Foley catheter.

       a.) Use a rubber band to occlude the tubing; clamps may perforate the tubing.

       b.) Cleanse the specimen port with an alcohol or iodophor wipe and aspirate the specimen with a 23 gauge needle and 5 ml syringe.

       c.) Take specimen to laboratory immediately.

       d.) Latex catheters reseal themselves if punctured at a 45° angle; Silastic catheters generally do not.

IV. Interpretation of culture results.

  A. In a clean-catch specimen, 100,000 col/ml of any organism is significant.

  B. In catheter specimens, greater than 1,000 col/ml of any organism is significant.

V. Symptoms of urinary tract infection.

  A. Acutely infected patient.

Pyelonephritis	Cystitis
back pain	urgency
fever	frequency
chills	dysuria
abdominal pain	incontinence
nausea	hematuria
	cloudy urine

  B. Chronically infected patient.

Pyelonephritis	Cystitis
low back pain	nocturia
easy fatigability	anorexia, weight loss
growth disturbances (in children)	

  C. Asymptomatic patient.

     1. Often found during a routine examination, especially in pregnancy.

2. May have had symptoms but not noticed them.

3. May see physician for symptoms of hypertension or its complications and physician finds the UTI.

VI. Common causes and prevention of urinary tract infections.

A. Dirty hands are a common cause of catheter-associated urinary tract infection.

1. Handling of any catheter or urine bag may contaminate with the infecting organisms.

2. The organisms infecting urine are motile and easily enter and may move upward within a contaminated system.

B. Open drainage systems cause infections: Systems that are either open by design or opened for irrigations or other reasons permit entry of microorganisms.

C. Prevention.

1. Wash hands after handling any urine bag or catheter.

2. All systems should be kept closed.

3. Irrigations should be by three-way catheter or not at all.

4. Avoid unnecessary changing of catheters and bags. (Silicone catheters may be preferable if long-term catheterization is anticipated.)

   a.) Evaluate the catheter by rolling it between your fingers; a sandy sensation indicates a need for change.

   b.) Observe the tubing; the buildup of sediment in it means there is probably the same buildup in the catheter; it is now time for a change.

5. Do not use Foley catheters solely for nursing convenience.

   a.) Insert a Foley only when absolutely necessary.

   b.) Once it is there, manipulate the system only when essential.

6. Keep all urine drainage bags below the level of the bladder but off the floor; do not permit sags or loops in drainage tubing.

7. Do not rely on commercial reflux valves. They are not fool-proof.

D. The immune-compromised or physically compromised patient is more likely to become infected.

1. Keep the patient well hydrated.

2. Discourage catheter placement in these patients.

     3. Do not put an infected patient with a Foley in a room with an uninfected catheterized patient.

VII. Intermittent self-catheterization.
    A. In the home, a clean procedure is adequate.
    B. In the hospital, it is a sterile procedure.
       1. Many hospital pathogens are resistant organisms that cause life-threatening infections.
       2. Hospitalized patients are usually compromised physically and are more likely to become infected.

VIII. Leg bags.
    A. Should be discouraged in the hospitalized patient.
    B. If leg bags are necessary, use a clean one daily.
    C. If unable to supply with a clean bag daily, the following should be done.
       1. Wash the bag with soap and water after use.
       2. Insert enough vinegar so all surfaces are covered.
       3. Before use again, discard vinegar, rinse bag thoroughly.
    D. Make sure catheter bag has a fresh sterile cap when not in use.
    E. Care must be taken so catheter is not rolled back and contaminated when detaching tubing.

T·E·S·T

1. List four elements that cause urine to be cloudy.
2. List three signs of urinary cystitis.
3. Describe the routes of infection from contaminated hands to bladder in a Foley-catheterized patient.
4. What is the minimum number of bacterial colonies indicating infection in a first morning clean-catch urine culture? In a catheter-urine culture?
5. What are two ways to detect calcium salts buildup in a Foley catheter?

A·N·S·W·E·R·S

1. Bacteria, white blood cells, red blood cells, and crystals may cloud urine.
2. Dysuria, frequency, incontinence, and nocturia are signs of cystitis.
3. Hands touching the outside of the Foley bag may contaminate the bag, subsequently the drainage tube and the urine in the bag. Bacteria can then migrate up the tube and into the bladder.
4. With a first morning clean-catch urine specimen, 100,000 bacterial colonies or more indicate infection. With a catheter-urine culture, 1,000 colonies indicate infection.
5. Roll catheter between fingers; there is a gritty or grainy sensation if salt deposits are present. Inspect transparent connecting tube for buildup of salts.

5

Wound care

Purpose

This wound care protocol is established to assist the nurse in the assessment and management of the surgical wound. The assessment must consider preoperative factors, the procedure performed, and present needs for surgical dressing care. Adequacy of management depends on careful assessment.

Learning objectives

o Know the four major nursing functions in post-op wound care.
o Identify five preoperative considerations in developing plans for post-op wound care.
o Recognize the intraoperative factors that influence wound healing.
o List the classes of surgical wounds.
o Name two types of surgical wounds.
o List the functions of a surgical dressing.

Behavioral objectives

o Select the dressing materials appropriate to the type of surgical wound.
o Recognize the signs and symptoms of an infected wound.
o Use aseptic technique in application of a surgical dressing.

Wound care

I. Nursing functions in wound care.
   A. Assess the patient.
   B. Select dressing materials.
   C. Change surgical dressing.
   D. Observe for complications with action as indicated.

II. Pre-op assessment of the patient.
   A. General health—observe for presence or absence of infection risk hazards, including the following.
      1. Extremes of age.
      2. Diabetes.
      3. Obesity.
      4. Immune depression.
      5. Active infection.
   B. Length of hospital stay pre-op should be noted.
   C. Skin preparation technique influences outcome.
      1. Shaving worst of available techniques because it creates tiny abrasions.
      2. Use of depilatory better than shaving, but can induce chemical dermatitis.
      3. Clipping best, but not widely used because it does not give a smooth operative field.
      4. Shower with antibacterial soap should be included.

III. Intraoperative risks.
   A. Type of procedure and wound affect expected infection rates.

Classification of surgical wounds	Infection rate
Clean	1.8 – 5.0%
Clean-contaminated	8.9 – 10.8%
Contaminated	16.3 – 21.5%
Dirty or infected	28.5 – 38.1%

   B. Length of procedure—the longer the procedure, the higher the expected infection incidence.
   C. Technique breaks expose wound to contamination.
   D. Complications, such as inadvertent opening of viscus, are important.

184

E. Foreign bodies placed in wound may provide nidus for infection.

F. Drains function both as foreign bodies and conduits for bacteria from without.

IV. Expected infection rate and post-op care techniques depend on wound types.

A. Closed wound, no drains, edges well-approximated.

B. Open wound, drain through incision or packed open.

V. Functions of a surgical dressing.

A. Dressing protects wound from contamination.

B. Protection of wound from trauma yields better healing.

C. Compression helps control bleeding at wound site.

D. Absorptive dressing wicks blood and drainage away from wound.

E. Immobilization is essential to healing.

F. Debridement occurs as necrotic material adheres to the dressing and is removed.

G. Application of medications can be accomplished.

H. Concealment of wound aids patient's and visitors' emotional health.

VI. Selection of dressing materials.

A. Air-occlusive dressing consists of nonporous materials, including tape, and may be used to contain medications at the wound site.

B. Nonocclusive dressing.

1. Most frequently used dressing material.

2. Facilitates air circulation.

3. Wicks drainage away from wound.

4. May be used in primary and/or secondary dressings.

C. Nonadhesive dressing.

1. Draining wounds require frequent dressing changes.

2. Open wounds may need many inspections and dressing changes.

3. Graft sites do not tolerate adhesives well.

D. Medicated dressings.

1. Medication may be applied to or incorporated in dressing.

Wound care

      2. Provides a technique for debridement with digestive enzymes.

      3. Allows topical treatment of infected wound with antibiotics.

  E. Taping techniques depend on goal.

      1. To secure dressing may require minimum tape.

      2. Air occlusion demands much taping.

      3. Multiple changes suggest need for alternative fixation technique.

VII. Aseptic technique in dressing change.

  A. Wash hands before and after procedure.

  B. Work from central area outward.

  C. Dress incision prior to drain site.

  D. Change entire dressing rather than reinforce it.

VIII. Observation of wound for complications.

  A. Types of complications.

      1. Infection is most frequent; its signs and symptoms are the following.

         a.) Inflammation.

         b.) Tenderness, pain.

         c.) Heat.

         d.) Swelling.

         e.) Purulent drainage.

      2. Hemorrhage.

      3. Dehiscence.

      4. Evisceration.

  B. Report complications to physician promptly.

  C. Chart the following on permanent record.

      1. Assessment.

      2. Treatments.

      3. Action taken.

T·E·S·T

---

1. What common surgical complication is increased in situations of immune suppression, preoperative hospital stay over three days, and use of shave prep 12 hours or more pre-op?
2. List five functions of a surgical dressing.
3. In what three general wound types may nonadhesive dressings be indicated?
4. List five signs at the wound site that suggest infection.

Answers are on page 188.

A·N·S·W·E·R·S

1. Each situation increases the possibility of a surgical wound infection.
2. Surgical dressings protect from contamination; protect from trauma; aid in compression, absorption, immobilization, and debridement; deliver medications; and conceal wounds.
3. Nonadhesive dressings are used for draining wounds, open wounds, and graft sites.
4. Inflammation, tenderness, heat, swelling and purulent drainage at the wound site suggest infection.

6

Tracheostomy

Purpose

Tracheostomy provides airway and access for suctioning the lower respiratory tract. But since it bypasses upper-airway protective structures, there is easy access for infection. The purpose of this section is to teach meticulous aseptic technique in placement, care, and culturing to lessen the frequency of infection.

Learning objectives

○ Know techniques of maintaining patient tracheostomy without introducing infection.

○ Identify possible late complications of tracheostomy.

Behavioral objectives

○ Employ good aseptic technique in care of tracheostomy.

○ Communicate to patient and family proper technique in handling tracheostomy.

Tracheostomy

I. Placement of tracheostomy.
   A. Several types of tubes, may be plastic or metal, cuffed or uncuffed (Figure 6-1, page 192).
   B. Best done in operating room aseptically.
   C. Tube is placed at second tracheal ring so tip remains above the carina.
      1. Test cuff before placement.
      2. Should be checked with X-ray.
   D. Have in patient's room suction apparatus and an extra tube in case original one is coughed out.

II. Early care of tracheostomy.
   A. Observe frequently for excessive bleeding. Inform physician if bleeding occurs.
   B. Be certain tube is securely tied in place.
   C. Observe for major subcutaneous air leaks. Signified by skin crepitus or respiratory embarrassment.
   D. Observe for esophageal leak into trachea, dyspnea. Latter may indicate placement is too low.
   E. Suction only when secretions are audible or visible.
      1. Use sterile technique.
      2. Discard disposables.
      3. Allay fears of patient.
      4. Use humidification to protect tracheal epithelium and prevent formation of hardened plugs of blood or secretions.
   F. Clean and dress the tracheostomy when soiled with blood or secretions. See below for technique.
      1. Keep mouth and throat clean.
      2. Position patient on side.
      3. Keep cuff inflated properly.

III. Late complications of tracheostomy.
   A. Major hemorrhage. Tube erodes into major cervical vessel. May be fatal.
   B. Injury to trachea, cartilage; injury to nerves of phonation.
   C. Infection (a common complication).
      1. Introduced through tracheostomy by aspiration.
      2. Signs indicating pneumonia: fever, purulent sputum, cough, new infiltrate on X-ray.

IV. Care of the tracheostomy.
  A. Materials (Figure 6-2, page 192).
    1. Suction equipment.
    2. Tracheostomy care kit.
    3. Sterile normal saline.
    4. Hydrogen peroxide.
    5. Sterile gloves, two pairs.
  B. Procedure.
    1. Explain procedure to the patient.
    2. Have all equipment at bedside.
    3. Wash hands and open kit using sterile technique.
    4. Pour solutions into proper containers in kit.
    5. Don sterile gloves.
    6. Remove inner cannula and place in hydrogen peroxide.
    7. Remove stoma dressing and discard properly.
    8. Instill 1 to 5 cc saline into trachea and suction.
    9. If gloves are soiled, put on fresh gloves.
    10. Clean inner cannula with brush and pipe cleaners.
    11. Rinse cannula in saline.
    12. Reinsert cannula and lock in place.
    13. Cleanse outer plate and skin around stoma. Apply prescribed ointment to skin.
    14. If tape on tracheostomy is soiled, replace. Have assistant hold tube in place.
    15. Replace dressing with lint-free dressing.
    16. Record procedure in chart. Chart quantity and color of secretions, skin status.
  C. Special precautions.
    1. Procedure should be done as ordered on new tracheostomy—usually q3-4h—and prn. After airway is established, q8h.
    2. A spare tracheal tube of same kind and size should always be placed at bedside.
    3. Obturators for disposable tracheal tubes may be discarded. Obturators for metal tracheal tubes are to be stored in a container at the bedside.
    4. Do not cut gauze for dressing, as loose patches may be aspirated. Do not use dressing that is not absorbent.

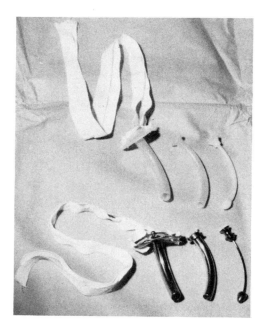

Figure 6-1: Various types of tracheostomy tubes.

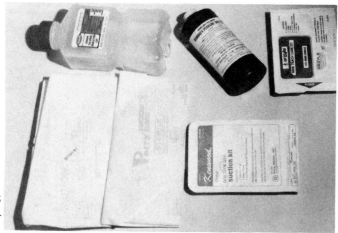

Figure 6-2: Materials for tracheostomy care.

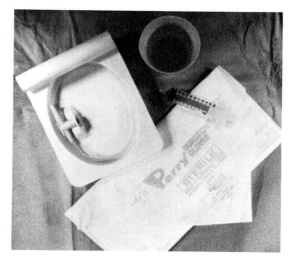

Figure 6-3:
Materials for suctioning
a tracheostomy.

V. Suctioning, a sterile procedure (Figure 6-3).
   A. Explain what is to be done.
   B. Wash hands, open suction kit.
   C. Don sterile gloves.
   D. Establish a sterile or clean field (latter is preferred).
   E. Attach a fresh suction tube.
   F. Pour sterile water into cup for rinsing tube.
   G. If secretions are tenacious, may use 1.5 cc sterile normal saline in trachea.
   H. Rinse entire system with sterile water after suctioning complete. Then discard all disposables.

T·E·S·T

---

1. List four early complications of tracheostomy.
2. List the four signs indicating pneumonia in a patient with a tracheostomy.
3. Ideally, tracheal suctioning is done on a _____.
   a. sterile field
   b. clean field
4. How long may the inner cannula be safely kept out of a tracheostomy if the patient is not on a ventilator?
5. How often should you suction a patient?

Answers are on page 194.

A·N·S·W·E·R·S

---

1. Bleeding, tracheoesophageal fistula, air leak, aspiration, copious secretions, coughing out tube are early complications of tracheostomy.
2. Unexplained fever, purulent secretions, predominant organism in smear and culture of secretions, and new infiltrate on chest X-ray lead to the assumption of pneumonia in a patient with a tracheostomy.
3. a. sterile field
4. Five minutes is the maximum period.
5. A patient should be suctioned whenever secretions are audible or visible.

7

Techniques for obtaining culture specimens

Purpose

The purpose of this section is to show the importance of culturing in infection control. Culturing proves presence or absence of bacteria and identifies those that are present. Culturing establishes the microbiologic safety of materials used in the hospital. Finally, it is a tool in the search for sources of infections—fomites, the inanimate environment, personnel, and other carriers.

Learning objectives

○ Understand the principles of culturing.

○ Know what materials are needed for each kind of specimen collection.

○ Know the steps of each collection procedure in their proper order.

Behavioral objectives

○ Deal effectively with difficult procedures or uncooperative patients.

○ Collect specimens in a manner that contributes to helpful laboratory testing.

Obtaining culture specimens

I. Classification of sites to be cultured.
   A. Normally sterile.
      1. Blood.
      2. Bladder urine.
      3. Spinal fluid.
      4. Other internal body fluids.
      5. Materials and supplies certified as sterile by the manufacturer or the central supply department.
   B. Normally colonized areas.
      1. Skin.
      2. Upper respiratory tract.
      3. Gastrointestinal tract.
      4. Female lower reproductive tract.
   C. Contaminated areas—normally sterile or colonized areas, which, because of temporary circumstances, acquire a noninfectious bacterial population.
      1. Trachea and large bronchi in an intubated patient.
      2. A decubitus ulcer, uninfected.
      3. A surgical wound during a clean surgical procedure.

II. Principles of culturing.
   A. Sterile areas—use strict sterile technique to avoid introducing external contaminants.
   B. Colonized areas—select for culture those areas that appear to harbor invasive pathogens: purulent areas on tonsils, purulence from deep within infected wounds, obviously purulent portions of a sputum specimen, and the like.
   C. Contaminated areas—remove contaminants as thoroughly as possible before culturing. Thus, if a patient has a grossly draining sinus tract, remove all superficial drainage before taking a culture. Likewise, if a patient has a middle ear infection with a ruptured tympanic membrane, clean the external canal thoroughly before aspirating for culture.
   D. Handling specimens.
      1. Culture specimens should be delivered promptly to the laboratory so that they may be placed in an environment that permits pathogens to grow but restricts overgrowth by contaminating bacteria.
      2. Specimens should not be permitted to dry.

3. Specimens for anaerobic culture must be protected from the air.

4. It is of obvious importance to prevent infectious materials from contacting skin or mucous membranes of the person collecting the culture specimen.

5. Specimens from patients in isolation should be properly labeled and protected.

III. Sputum for culture.
   A. General considerations.
      1. Oral contaminants can negate value of specimen.
      2. Rapid growth of contaminants occurs at room temperature.
      3. Principles of specimen collection.
         a.) Collect in early a.m.
         b.) Collect at least 15 ml.
         c.) Collect at least three specimens.
      4. Note on requisition whatever antibiotics patient is receiving.
      5. Check requisition to see that suspected infectious diagnosis is noted.
   B. Cooperative conscious patient with productive cough.
      1. Materials: Toothbrush, dentifrice, mouthwash, tissues, sterile sputum cup, and tap water (Figure 7-1).

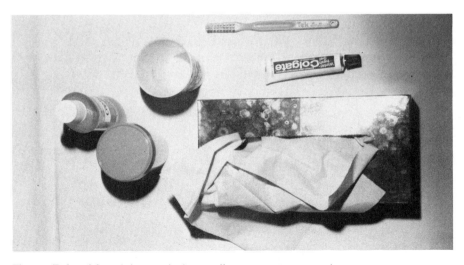

Figure 7-1: Materials needed to collect a sputum specimen.

Obtaining culture specimens

    2. Procedure.
- a.) Patient brushes teeth, rinses mouth, gargles with mouthwash, and rinses again three times with water.
- b.) After deep cough, patient expectorates into sterile sputum cup.
- c.) Double-bag and label isolated patient's specimen.
- d.) Deliver specimen to laboratory promptly.
- e.) Note in chart color, amount, consistency, and odor of specimens.

C. Cooperative conscious patient with nonproductive cough.
    1. Materials: Toothbrush, dentifrice, mouthwash, ultrasonic nebulizer, sterile normal saline (on M.D. order), sterile sputum cup, and tap water.
    2. Procedure.
- a.) Patient brushes teeth, rinses mouth, gargles with mouthwash, and rinses again three times with water.
- b.) Deliver normal saline by nebulization for 10 minutes.
- c.) Patient rinses mouth once.
- d.) Have patient expectorate into cup after deep cough.
- e.) Double-bag and label isolated patient's specimen.
- f.) Deliver specimen to laboratory promptly.
- g.) Note in chart color, amount, consistency, and odor of specimen.

D. Uncooperative, conscious patient.
    1. Materials: Assistants and/or restraints as required, 1 pair clean gloves, Lukens trap, suction catheter and vacuum source, water soluble lubricant, and clean drape.
    2. Procedure.
- a.) Obtain M.D. order, explain procedure to patient or guardian.
- b.) Restrain patient if necessary (later document need for restraint).
- c.) Put on gloves.
- d.) Assemble suction catheter and Lukens trap on clean drape.
- e.) Lubricate catheter tip.
- f.) Insert through naris, pass into trachea when patient inhales.

g.) Suction; if nothing comes, instill 5 cc normal saline through catheter and suction again.

h.) Double-bag and label isolated patient's specimen.

i.) Deliver specimen to laboratory promptly.

j.) Note in chart color, amount, consistency, and odor of specimen.

E. Unconscious patient: Same materials and procedure as for conscious uncooperative patient, except restraints are unnecessary.

F. Intubated patient.

1. Materials: Lukens trap, suction kit, saline without preservative, sterile cup.

2. Procedure.

a.) Use sterile procedure.

b.) Suction from trachea into Lukens trap.

c.) If necessary, rinse suction catheter into trap, using saline in sterile cup.

d.) Double-bag and label isolated patient's specimen.

e.) Deliver specimen to laboratory promptly.

f.) Note in chart color, amount, consistency, and odor of specimen.

IV. Urine for culture.

A. General considerations.

1. Quantity of contamination is proportionate to improper techniques.

2. Organisms double in specimen each 45 minutes.

3. Only first a.m. urines should be collected for clean-catch urine specimens.

4. Colony-forming units in excess of 100,000/ml constitutes infection, except for *Staphylococcus* and *Candida,* of which an excess of 10,000/ml constitutes infection, and a specimen collected from a catheter, in which case anything in excess of 1000/ml signifies infection.

5. Almost all UTIs are single-organism infections. Common exceptions are patients with indwelling catheters or GU fistulas.

6. A repeat (confirmation) urine for culture is necessary in women when clean-catch technique is used to diagnose

Obtaining culture specimens

UTI. A single midstream clean-catch urine for culture from a woman is only 75 to 85 percent accurate. Therefore, in many situations a single straight catheter specimen may be preferable and ordered by the physician.

B. Clean-catch specimen from an adult cooperative female (cooperative patient can perform entire procedure after instruction).
1. Materials: cleaning material (sudsing soap and tap water) for urethral orifice, sterile specimen cup.
2. Procedure.
   a.) Specimen cup should be open before beginning.
   b.) Separate and hold apart labia during procedure.
   c.) Wash urethral orifice thoroughly with soap.
   d.) Rinse well with tap water.
   e.) Have patient begin to urinate into toilet or bedpan. Without stopping the stream, collect the middle portion in the specimen cup.
   f.) Deliver promptly to the laboratory or place in ice bath. (Warm articles in a refrigerator develop an insulating layer of stationary air that retards cooling. Therefore, if cooling is necessary, use an ice bath.)

C. Clean-catch specimen from an adult cooperative male (cooperative patient can perform entire procedure after instructions).
1. Materials: cleaning material (sudsing soap and tap water) for glans, sterile specimen cup.
2. Procedure.
   a.) Open specimen cup before beginning procedure.
   b.) Retract foreskin.
   c.) Wash glans thoroughly with soap.
   d.) Rinse well with tap water.
   e.) Have patient start urine stream and, without stopping stream, collect middle portion in the specimen cup.
   f.) Deliver promptly to the laboratory or place in ice bath.

D. Uncooperative, unconscious, or bedridden (female) patient (or any patient, at doctor's discretion).
1. Materials: straight sterile catheter, antibacterial soap, specimen cup, assistant (optional).

2. Procedure.

    a.) Patient must be well hydrated one hour prior to catheterization.

    b.) Sterile procedure on a sterile field.

    c.) Place catheter into bladder.

    d.) Discard the first and last portion of the urine, collect the middle 10 to 25 ml in the specimen cup.

    e.) Deliver promptly to the laboratory or place in ice bath.

E. Uncooperative child: Use straight catheterization or ask physician about suprapubic aspiration of bladder urine (not a nursing procedure).

F. A Foley-catheterized patient.

1. Materials: Alcohol, sponge, sterile 3 to 5 cc syringe, 23-g needle, sterile specimen cup.

2. Procedure.

    a.) Obstruct tubing for 10 to 15 minutes with a rubber band, not a clamp (Figure 7-2).

    b.) If catheter does not have a special port, cleanse a short segment of rubber tubing with alcohol, then puncture tubing at an acute angle, with the needle and syringe distal to the inflation port. Fill syringe.

    c.) Send specimen in syringe immediately to laboratory or place in sterile specimen cup and deliver immediately to laboratory or place in ice bath.

V. Other cultures.

A. Throat culture.

1. Materials: Two calcium alginate or dacron culture swabs, tongue blade, light (Figure 7-3), assistant (optional).

2. Procedure.

    a.) Inspect throat, using light and tongue blade.

    b.) Rub area of purulence or inflammation (tonsils or pharynx) with swab; don't touch tongue.

    c.) One swab per tonsil.

    d.) Place in container and send to laboratory.

B. Wound culture.

1. Materials: gloves (one pair sterile, one pair clean), material to replace dressing, paper bag, 4 × 4s, aerobic culture swabs, anaerobic container or sterile 5 cc syringe, 22-g needle, saline for irrigation.

Obtaining culture specimens

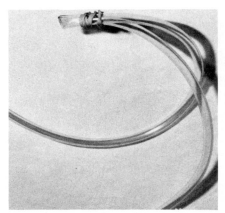

Figure 7-2: Catheter tube should be obstructed with a rubber band.

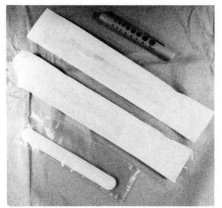

Figure 7-3: Materials needed to collect specimen from throat.

2. Procedure.
   a.) Wash hands, put on clean gloves.
   b.) Remove dressing and place in paper bag.
   c.) Cleanse around the wound, using no-touch technique; remove all visible secretions.
   d.) Aspirate drainage from the wound with the syringe or swab from depths of wound.
   e.) If swabs are used, place one in anaerobic transport medium. If a syringe is used, express any air from the syringe, attach needle, and cap the needle with a rubber stopper.

C. Blood culture.
   1. General considerations.
      a.) Quality of skin preparation is crucial to limiting contamination.
      b.) Blood is a sterile fluid; therefore, isolation of a microorganism is strong evidence for disease.
      c.) Bacteremia peaks one-half to one hour before fever.
   2. Materials: Tourniquet, aerobic and anaerobic culture bottles, sterile syringe (or vacuum tube) and two 22-g needles, iodophor skin prep swabs, and alcohol swabs.

202

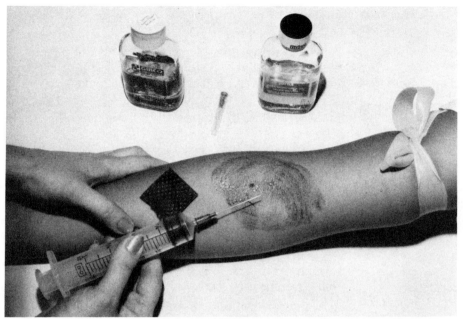

Figure 7-4:   Collecting a blood specimen.

3. Procedure (Figure 7-4).
   a.) Apply tourniquet to upper arm.
   b.) Locate a prominent vein.
   c.) Prep the area over the vein, using an expanding circular motion. Use two iodophor swabs.
   d.) Permit iodophor to remain at least four minutes.
   e.) Prep your fingertip if you must touch skin site.
   f.) Aseptically aspirate 10 cc of blood.
   g.) Change needles.
   h.) Deliver 5 cc blood to each bottle without introducing air.
   i.) Follow instructions on bottle for venting aerobic bottle.
   j.) Wipe iodophor off patient's skin with alcohol swab.
   k.) Deliver culture bottles to laboratory.
   l.) If other site—artery, central venous line, femoral vein—must be used for culture, be certain to note this on the requisition.

Obtaining culture specimens

D. Nasopharyngeal swab.
  1. General considerations.
      a.) This is an uncomfortable procedure for the patient. You may need an assistant for collecting a specimen from a small child. Reassure adult patients.
      b.) Wooden-handled swabs should not be used. Use a fine-wire swab with dacron, such as is used for urethral cultures.
  2. Materials: Wire with dacron or calcium alginate urethral swab, sterile container, and otoscope with nasal speculum; an assistant is optional.
  3. Procedure.
      a.) Inspect both nares with the otoscope to select one that is not occluded.
      b.) While the patient is supine and breathing deeply through his mouth, insert the swab through one naris until it touches the posterior pharynx.
      c.) Twist the swab, then withdraw it.
      d.) Place in container and deliver promptly to the laboratory.

E. Nasal cultures.
  1. Purpose: To detect carriers of *Staphylococcus, Pseudomonas,* and perhaps *Candida.*
  2. Materials: wooden stick with dacron culture swab, container.
  3. Procedure.
      a.) Ask patient to lie supine.
      b.) Insert the swab no more than 1 cm into naris and swab in a circular motion.
      c.) Place in container and deliver promptly to laboratory.

F. Vaginal cultures.
  1. General considerations.
      a.) The vagina is heavily populated with bacteria. Therefore, only isolation of recognized pathogens is significant.
      b.) The normal flora grows rapidly and will obscure pathogens if culture specimen is mishandled.
  2. Materials: Clean gloves, wooden stick with dacron culture swabs, container, and good light.

3. Procedure.

    a.) Don gloves.

    b.) Have patient lie in lithotomy position.

    c.) Hold the labia apart with one hand and insert swab 2 to 3 cm under good visualization.

    d.) Swab in a circular motion.

    e.) Place swab in container.

    f.) Deliver promptly to laboratory.

G. Cervical culture.

  1. General considerations.

    a.) Must avoid contamination with vaginal flora.

    b.) The cervical mucus plug should not be cultured.

    c.) Culture should be from the endocervix.

  2. Materials: gloves, speculum, good light source (gooseneck lamp), three sterile dacron swabs, culture container, Thayer-Martin or Transgrow medium.

  3. Procedure.

    a.) Don gloves, position light.

    b.) Have patient lie in lithotomy position.

    c.) Insert speculum to visualize cervix.

    d.) With one swab, remove any secretions from the speculum. Discard.

    e.) With the second swab, remove the mucus plug from the cervix. Discard.

    f.) Insert the third swab 1 to 2 cm into the cervical canal, rotate, remove.

    g.) Place swab in container and send immediately to laboratory.

    h.) If gonococcus is being sought, inoculate a Thayer-Martin or Transgrow bottle immediately, then send the swab to the laboratory. Medium should be prewarmed and placed in CO_2 atmosphere as soon as it is inoculated.

H. Rectal swab.

  1. General considerations.

    a.) One value of a rectal swab is in getting material from the perirectal tissues to culture for *Shigella,* not stool, which would yield *Salmonella.*

        b.) Rectal swabs may be useful in epidemiological surveys.

2. Materials: gloves, light source, large calcium alginate or dacron swab.

3. Procedure.

    a.) Have patient lie on his side with legs flexed at the hips or have him bend over a table.

    b.) Adjust light.

    c.) Don gloves.

    d.) Spread buttocks to visualize anus.

    e.) Gently insert swab about 2 to 3 cm (1 to 2 in infants); swab all four quadrants.

    f.) Swab should be placed immediately in culture medium.

    g.) For stool culture, send a walnut-sized piece of fresh stool in a sterile container.

I. Eye cultures.

1. General considerations.

    a.) Swabs must be taken before topical anesthetics are applied to avoid dilution or antibacterial preservative action.

    b.) If anesthetics have been used, the doctor should collect corneal scrapings.

    c.) In swabbing the conjunctiva, the cornea must not be touched.

2. Procedure.

    a.) Carefully evert the lower lid with a gloved hand. Gloves should be free of talc.

    b.) Gently swab the everted conjunctiva, collecting as much material as possible.

    c.) Deliver immediately to laboratory for smear and culture.

J. Ear cultures.

1. Swabs of material from the canal are inadequate for diagnosis of middle ear infection.

2. Tympanocentesis must be performed by the doctor.

3. Cultures for otitis externa may be collected by swabbing the surface gently with an alginate swab.

K. Intravascular line cultures.

1. General considerations.

       a.) A technique for semiquantitative assessment of results is necessary.

       b.) Any skin surface purulence must be removed prior to pulling the line.

  2. Materials: Sterile gloves, alcohol swabs, sterile scissors, sterile forceps, suture removal set, blood agar culture plate, tube of thioglycollate broth, sterile drape.

  3. Procedure.

       a.) Wash hands.

       b.) Don gloves, open sterile drape.

       c.) Remove dressings.

       d.) Carefully cleanse around puncture site with alcohol swab.

       e.) Remove catheter, applying pressure over site after removal. Put catheter on sterile drape.

       f.) With sterile scissors, cut off the inner three inches of the catheter, place it on one side of the agar plate, and with the forceps roll it once to the other side.

       g.) Place the catheter tip in a tube of thioglycollate broth.

       h.) Deliver plate and broth to bacteriology.

L. Culturing nonhuman sources.

  1. General considerations.

       a.) Employed for epidemiologic purposes.

       b.) Variety of materials cultured: surfaces, instruments, supplies, IV fluids. Each requires specific techniques.

       c.) Should consult laboratory director and epidemiologist for specific details.

  2. Procedure for culturing flat surfaces.

       a.) With a dry sterile swab, swab in two directions over a $2'' \times 2''$ area.

       b.) Transfer swab to a blood agar plate, and swab the plate in two directions over its entire surface and also roll the swab.

  3. Procedure for culturing tubing.

       a.) Deliver 10 ml of culture broth into tubing and run it back and forth through the middle two-thirds of the tubing.

       b.) Aseptically pour the broth into a sterile specimen cup.

       c.) Deliver to laboratory for quantitative culture.

4. Procedure for evaluating air.
   a.) Place four to six open blood agar plates face up on surfaces and permit organisms to fall on them for 15 minutes.
   b.) Repeat study at time of suspected low and high contamination.
5. Procedure for culturing IV fluids.
   a.) The laboratory should perform this analysis, using a standard water-testing micropore filter and an adequate volume of the fluid in question.
   b.) This procedure is an important component of workup of fever occurring in a patient receiving parenteral hyperalimentation fluids. See Chapter 12 for details.
6. Procedure for culturing hands.
   a.) Place 100 ml sterile culture broth in a plastic bag.
   b.) Have person insert hand into broth and vigorously stir the broth with his hand.
   c.) Ask laboratory to do quantitative and qualitative culture on the broth.

T·E·S·T

1. Give an example of each and list the three categories of sites from which cultures are taken.
2. True/False
   A.＿＿ The nasopharynx should be cultured with flexible wire culture swab.
   B.＿＿ Blood cultures drawn from IV lines are of no value.
   C.＿＿ A rectal swab is needed to diagnose *Shigella*. A stool specimen is needed for *Salmonella*.
   D.＿＿ IV catheters may be adequately cultured by simply immersing the catheter tip in culture broth.
   E.＿＿ Two clean-catch urine cultures are necessary to establish urinary infection in a woman.

A·N·S·W·E·R·S

1. **Category**   **Example**
   Sterile   Blood
   Colonized   Throat
   Contaminated   Decubitus ulcer

2. True/False
   A. True
   B. False
   C. True
   D. False
   E. True

8

Hepatitis A

Purpose

This section reviews the epidemiology, mode of transmission, and symptomatology of hepatitis A. Technique for control in the hospital environment is described.

Learning objectives

○ Recognize the symptoms of hepatitis A.

○ Know the mode of spread and most common sources of hepatitis A infection.

○ Understand what constitutes an exposure to hepatitis A and the appropriate prophylaxis.

Behavioral objectives

○ Establish proper control measures for the hospitalized patient with hepatitis A.

○ Provide appropriate teaching for the infected patient.

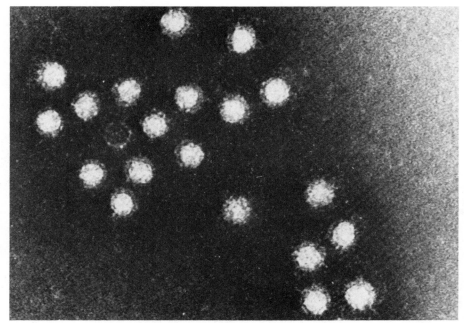

Figure 8-1: *Electron micrograph of hepatitis A viruses. Reproduced with permission of Cutter Biologicals.*

I. The virus.

    A. Identifiable by electron microscopy (Figure 8-1).

    B. Virus is sphere-shaped, 27 nm long, which is smaller than hepatitis B virus.

    C. Abbreviation for it is HAV.

II. Epidemiology.

    A. Seasonal variation.

        1. Fall to winter is most common.

        2. Since 1966, no significant seasonal changes in incidence in U.S.

    B. Incidence.

        1. Greatest in countries with poor sanitation.

            a.) Travelers to Far East, South America, or any underdeveloped area should receive prophylaxis.

            b.) Travelers should avoid tap water, fresh produce, and ice.

2. From 30 to 40 percent of U.S. population and up to 80 percent of adults have antibody to hepatitis A.

    a.) Many cases are undiagnosed.

    b.) Diagnosis may be missed due to other disorders accompanied by liver dysfunction, such as the following.

       (1). Alcoholism.

       (2.) Gallbladder disease.

       (3.) Drug-induced hepatitis.

       (4.) Anesthesia-induced hepatitis.

C. Natural reservoirs.

    1. Asymptomatic acute cases or carriers (rare).

    2. Institutions.

       a.) Schools for mentally handicapped children.

       b.) Day-care centers.

    3. Contaminated water supplies.

III. Mode of transmission.

A. Human feces-contaminated food/water.

    1. Water supply contaminated by human waste.

    2. Milk.

    3. Raw oysters.

    4. Green salad, other food contaminated by carriers or, in some countries, human fertilizer.

    5. Foods, such as bakery items, that are handled after cooking.

B. School outbreaks, especially in nursery/primary grades.

    1. Poor hygienic practices of children spread hepatitis among students. It is often asymptomatic.

    2. Failure of family members to wash hands after contact with contaminated items from students spreads disease to the remainder of the family.

C. Infectious body excretions/secretions.

    1. Patient's blood (unusual source).

    2. Patient's urine.

    3. Patient's stool (most common source).

    4. Patient's saliva (questionable source; presence of virus may be due to bleeding from gums).

Hepatitis

     5. Maximum communicability during incubation period prior to symptoms.

IV. Clinical picture.

  A. Incubation period 10 to 50 days, average 21 to 35.

  B. Signs and symptoms. (There may be prodromal migratory arthralgias early in the incubation period.)
1. Fever up to 104°F.
2. Malaise.
3. Anorexia, early loss of taste for cigarettes.
4. Abdominal discomfort.
5. Nausea, vomiting.
6. Jaundice, tea-colored urine, clay-colored stool.
7. Elevated liver enzymes.

  C. Diagnosis.
1. Rule out other forms of hepatitis.
   a.) Negative HBsAg and anti-HBc helpful.
   b.) Positive anti-HBsAg compatible; may only indicate remote infection with hepatitis B.
   c.) No history of receiving blood products in last six months.
   d.) No other pathologic process causative of liver pathology, such as infectious mononucleosis, leptospirosis, yellow fever, toxoplasmosis.
2. RIA for hepatitis A virus antibody (anti-HAV).
   a.) Rising titer of anti-HAV during illness (four-fold rise in titer is diagnostic).
   b.) Significant titer of IgM antibody to HAV is evidence for recent infection.

  D. Clinical course.

1. Moderate illness lasting one to two weeks.
2. May be disabling for several months, though this is unusual.
3. Recovery without sequelae or recurrences.
4. Mortality and chronicity are rare.

214

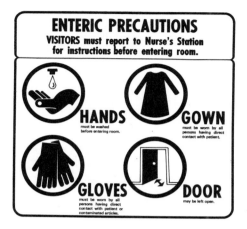

ENTERIC PRECAUTIONS
VISITORS must report to Nurse's Station
for instructions before entering room.

HANDS
must be washed
before entering room.

GOWN
must be worn by all
persons having direct
contact with patient.

GLOVES
must be worn by all
persons having direct
contact with patient or
contaminated articles.

DOOR
may be left open.

Figure 8-2: Enteric precautions are used in cases of hepatitis A infection. (Courtesy, St. Joseph's Hospital, Tampa.)

V. Isolation precautions.
   A. Enteric precautions (Figure 8-2).
      1. Required only for fecally incontinent.
      2. Private room desirable.
   B. Excretion precautions.
      1. Used for cooperative and educable patient.
      2. Double room is permissible.
      3. Gloves are worn for handling all secretions and excretions and to handle tubes or instruments entering intestinal tract.
      4. May share toilet facilities if continent and cooperative.

VI. Patient teaching.
   A. Review basic hygiene, especially hand washing after using toilet facilities.
   B. Traffic control.
      1. Should not use public restrooms in the hospital.
      2. Should not use public eating facilities in the hospital.

VII. Prophylaxis.
   A. Usually required only for family members or those with oral exposure to patient's body secretions or excretions.
   B. Immune serum globulin 0.03 ml/kg by body weight within seven days of exposure, given IM.
   C. Effective up to three months.

Hepatitis B

Purpose

This section reviews the epidemiology, mode of transmission, and symptomatology of hepatitis B. New terminology is defined. Patient teaching concepts for both hospitalized patients and patients in a community or home environment are presented.

Learning objectives

○ Know the mode of spread and most common source of hepatitis B.

○ Define HBV, HBsAg, and anti-HBs.

○ State the incubation period and symptoms of hepatitis B.

○ Understand the most common ways hospital personnel may acquire hepatitis B and what the appropriate prophylaxis is.

○ Differentiate between HBV antibodies and HBV antigens and know the significance when either are identified in a patient's blood.

Behavioral objectives

○ Establish the proper control measures for the hospitalized patient with hepatitis B.

○ Instruct the patient who is HBsAg positive in proper hygiene and health practices to prevent spread of HBV in the community or home environment.

I. The virus (referred to as Dane particle).

   A. Observable by electron microscopy (Figure 8-3).

   B. Virus size is 45 nm. Looks like a herpesvirus.

   C. Abbreviation for it is HBV.

II. Epidemiology.

   A. No seasonal variation.

   B. Incidence.

      1. Greatest between ages 15 and 29, more prone are hemophiliacs, IV drug abusers, male homosexuals, dialysis patients.

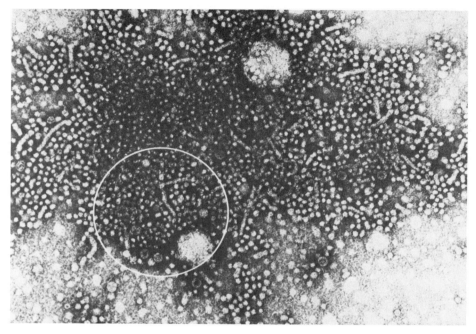

Figure 8-3: *Electron micrograph of hepatitis B virus and surface antigen. (Reproduced with permission of Cutter Biologicals.)*

    2. Health-care workers have at least two times the risk of community members.

        a.) Departments where risk of exposure to hepatitis B is high.

            (1.) Operating room.

            (2.) Intensive care units.

            (3.) Dialysis units.

            (4.) Renal wards.

            (5.) Hematology/oncology wards.

            (6.) Dental departments.

            (7.) Immunology laboratories.

        b.) Personnel at risk.

            (1.) Oral surgeons.

            (2.) Pathologists.

            (3.) Surgeons.

            (4.) Anesthetists.

            (5.) Nephrologists.

(6.) Anyone who draws blood or handles blood or blood products.

(7.) Laboratory workers.

(8.) All personnel with direct patient contact working in a high-risk department.

(9.) Highest rates of hepatitis B are among technicians and practical nurses.

3. From seven to 10 percent of hepatitis cases transmitted by blood or blood products are cases of hepatitis B. Use of blood from commercial donors increases risk to patient.

4. Underdeveloped countries have a high incidence of hepatitis B.

a.) Refugees entering the U.S. comprise a new source of hepatitis B.

b.) Some travelers may need immunoprophylaxis, and all should use care in choice of beverages and foods.

III. Mode of transmission.

A. Contaminated food and water are uncommon sources.

B. Infused contaminated blood products.

C. Infectious body excretions and secretions.

1. Blood and blood products.

a.) Serous wound drainage.

b.) Menstrual secretions.

2. Urine.

3. Semen and vaginal secretions.

4. Tears.

5. Saliva.

6. Perspiration.

D. Contaminated materials can infect by parenteral inoculation or by contact with broken skin or intact mucous membranes.

E. Infants born to mothers with hepatitis B may have congenital or neonatal hepatitis B. They have high frequency of carrier state and subsequent liver disorders.

IV. Clinical picture.

A. Incubation period is six weeks to six months (mean 60 days).

B. Signs and symptoms.

1. Urticaria and/or arthralgia are common prodromal symptoms.
2. Malaise.
3. Anorexia, loss of taste for cigarettes variable.
4. Vomiting is not as prominent as with hepatitis A.
5. Fatigue.
6. Mental depression.
7. Elevated liver enzymes.
8. Icterus (anicteric disease two to three times more common).
9. Dark urine.
10. Light stools.

C. Diagnosis.
   1. RIA or EIA for hepatitis B surface antigen (HBsAg).
     a.) Coating on outer surface of virus.
     b.) Presence in blood indicates infectivity.
   2. RIA or EIA for hepatitis B antibody (anti-HBs, anti-HBc).
     a.) Presence of anti-HBs indicates past infection, protection from hepatitis B.
     b.) Anti-HBc rises early in disease; may persist for many years.
       (1.) May have had known active disease.
       (2.) May have had unknown, undiagnosed disease.
       (3.) May have had many mini-exposures and developed antibody, which often occurs in persons working in high-risk areas.
       (4.) Immunity from injected anti-HBs usually does not last unless person is challenged and develops active infection.
       (5.) Four-fold rise in titer indicates recent hepatitis B.
       (6.) Anti-HBs may be only positive test early in recovery.
   3. Liver function tests—elevated (SGOT, SGPT, alkaline phosphatase, GGTP, LDH).
   4. Symptoms are not diagnostic.
   5. History may be very helpful.
     a.) Exposure to known hepatitis B.

       b.) Received blood products in last six months.

       c.) Drug addiction, homosexuality, health-care worker.

D. Clinical course.
  1. May be mild or severe acute disease or chronic disease; rarely is it fulminant and fatal.
     a.) Individual's defense mechanisms may alter severity of disease.
     b.) How acquired may be significant factor in disease severity.
  2. Carrier state.
     a.) Five to 10 percent become HBsAg carriers. State lasts a few weeks to a lifetime.
     b.) Some patients very likely to be carriers.
       (1.) Renal transplant patients.
       (2.) Dialysis patients.
       (3.) Immunosuppressed patients.
       (4.) Congenitally infected.
  3. Chronic persistent hepatitis.
     a.) Disease has been present six or more months.
     b.) Asymptomatic.
     c.) Positive HBsAg.
     d.) Positive anti-HBc.
     e.) If HBeAg or DNA polymerase positive, patient has high risk of aggressive disease and is infectious.
  4. Chronic aggressive hepatitis.
     a.) Disease has been present six or more months.
     b.) Symptoms of liver necrosis may occur.
     c.) Positive HBsAg.
     d.) Positive anti-HBc.
     e.) Prognosis worse and infectiousness higher if HBeAg or DNA polymerase is positive.
  5. Fulminant viral hepatitis.
     a.) Acute, frequently fatal (mortality is 70 percent).
     b.) Not necessarily preceded by chronic aggressive hepatitis.
     c.) Signs of liver failure predominate.

V. Isolation and precautions.
   A. Enteric precautions (see Figure 8-2, page 215) and blood precautions (see Figure 8-6, page 226).
      1. Incontinent, uncooperative, uneducable patients and children.
      2. Private room desirable.
      3. May be walked in hall but not permitted to use public restrooms or eating facilities in hospital.
      4. Label laboratory specimens "Hepatitis."
      5. Infected children should not share toys.
   B. Secretion and blood precautions.
      1. Educable and cooperative patient.
      2. Personnel wear gloves for handling any secretion or excretion-contaminated items or linen.
      3. May walk in hall but not permitted to use public restrooms or eating facilities.
      4. Infected children should not share toys.
      5. Label laboratory specimens "Hepatitis."
   C. Blood precautions.
      1. Utilized for HBsAg carriers.
      2. Wear gloves for all blood drawing, venipuncture, and the like.
      3. Use disposable needles and syringes and dispose of in an impervious container.
      4. Label all laboratory specimens "Hepatitis."

VI. Patient teaching.
   A. Review basic hygiene/health practices.
      1. Hands must be washed after using toilet facilities.
      2. There must be no sharing of towels, razors, toothbrushes, emery boards, or any personal-care items.
      3. Warn family members about eating from or drinking from patient's used food or beverage containers.
      4. If cooking for a family, use a separate dish and utensil to taste foods.
      5. Do not pick at blemishes, sores, and the like.
         a.) Blood is highly infectious.
         b.) Places others at risk.

      6. Take care with menstrual secretions.

        a.) Use plastic bags to discard sanitary napkins.

        b.) Tampons may be used.

      7. Disease may be sexually transmitted to consort.

      8. Discuss hepatitis B vaccine.

B. Dishware.

    1. May use disposable dishware.

    2. May rinse dishware with household bleach and then wash as usual.

    3. May use a dishwasher that reaches 189°F.

      a.) With dishwasher's built-in heater (if it has one) boosting water temperature to 189°F.

      b.) Or with hot water heater set that high.

C. Use of toilet facilities.

    1. Decontaminate with bleach after use.

    2. Or use separate bathroom.

D. Sexual activity: alternative precautions.

    1. Abstinence is totally protective against transmission.

    2. Use of condom is highly effective.

    3. HBIG for partner—proof of effectiveness incomplete.

    4. HBIG for partner and use condom.

    5. ISG for partner—proof of effectiveness incomplete.

    6. ISG for partner and use condom—unproven.

    7. Hepatitis B vaccine very effective.

    8. No precautions.

      a.) Few patients feel well enough to have sexual activity anyway.

      b.) Partner may have been previously exposed, in which case prophylaxis will be of no benefit.

E. Decontamination of clothing soiled by blood, secretions, or excretions.

    1. Colorfast cotton, linen, rayon, nylon, dacron, or orlon may be machine-washed.

      a.) Separate from family items.

      b.) Use household bleach (5.25 percent sodium hypochlorite) with laundry detergent and hot water.

2. Hand-washable items should be soaked 10 minutes in hot water to which detergent and bleach (two tbsp per gallon) have been added.

3. Boilable fabrics may be boiled 30 minutes and then laundered.

F. Decontamination of hard surfaces.

1. Use household bleach.

2. Immersible items may be boiled 30 minutes.

VII. Personnel safety.

A. Protection while delivering patient care.

1. Wear gloves whenever handling blood or blood products and while performing venipunctures or similar procedures.

2. Wear a gown to protect attire if blood contamination of clothing is a possibility.

3. Report any personal injury or exposure involving HBsAg secretions, excretions, or blood or blood products.

a.) Blood in eye, nose, or any mucous membrane surface.

b.) Cut or scratch caused by blood-contaminated item.

c.) Blood entering an existing cut, scratch, and the like.

d.) Other secretions or excretions of HBsAg-infected patient have entered the body.

(1.) Sharing a beverage or food.

(2.) Sexual intercourse.

(3.) Touching an open wound or scratch.

4. Obtain appropriate prophylaxis.

a.) Hepatitis B immune globulin (anti-HBs)

(1.) High HBV antibody titer.

(2.) Expensive ($75 to $200 per dose).

(3.) Used only for proven HBsAg blood exposures.

(4.) One dose at time of exposure and repeat in 30 days.

(5.) Questionable effectiveness.

(6.) Can extend incubation period to greater than eight months.

b.) Immune serum globulin (ISG).

(1.) All ISG has antibody for HBV.

        (2.) One dose at time of exposure and repeat in 30 days.

        (3.) Less effective than anti-HBs.

    c.) Immunization with hepatitis B vaccine.

B. Keeping the work environment safe.
1. Handle all blood or blood products as if infected.
2. Place all soiled needles and sharp items in an impervious container.
    a.) Never recap used needles.
    b.) Never break used needles.
    c.) Discard used IV piggyback needles immediately.
3. Clean up blood spills.
    a.) Wear gloves.
    b.) Wipe up spills with a disposable towel or rag.
    c.) Dispose of rag in impervious bag.
    d.) Flood area with virucidal agent.
    e.) Wipe up agent with a disposable towel or rag and discard.
    f.) Place gloves in bag.
    g.) Seal and discard bag.
4. Immunize high-risk personnel.

VIII. Hepatitis B during pregnancy, neonatal period, and infancy.
A. Transmission of disease.
1. Transplacental transmission is difficult to distinguish from HBV exposure at or near time of delivery.
    a.) Prior to third trimester, virus can cause fetal abnormalities.
    b.) Actual mode of intrauterine transmission is uncertain.
2. Modes of transmission at or near birth.
    a.) Maternal blood.
    b.) Amniotic fluid.
    c.) Menstrual blood.
    d.) Breast milk.
    e.) Saliva.
B. Frequency of disease in infants.
1. Higher in those with chronic carrier mothers.

2. Higher in those with an acutely ill mother.
C. HBV in neonates.
   1. More often premature.
   2. Frequently become chronic carriers.
   3. High frequency of hepatocellular carcinoma.

Non-A, non-B hepatitis

Purpose
This section defines non-A, non-B hepatitis, reviews its epidemiology, mode of transmission, symptomatology, and the steps to take in preventing its occurrence and spread in the hospital.

Learning objectives
○ Know the rate of occurrence of non-A, non-B hepatitis in transfused patients.
○ List the blood products most often responsible for transmission of non-A, non-B hepatitis.
○ Describe the proper method of cleaning up blood spilled from an infected patient and list the germicides active against non-A, non-B hepatitis.
○ List three types of exposure to an infected patient that would require prophylaxis to prevent acquiring the disease.

Behavioral objectives
○ Place the non-A, non-B hepatitis patient in proper precautions.
○ Alert nursing and hospital personnel to patients with a high risk of the disease.
○ Clean up a blood spill from an infected patient and decontaminate the spill area.

Hepatitis

I. The virus.
  A. Viral particle has not been identified.
  B. That recurrence not uncommon is evidence for more than one form.

II. Epidemiology.
  A. Represents 80 to 90 percent of transfusion-associated hepatitis.
  B. Most commonly associated with history of receiving a transfusion of a blood product.

III. Mode of transmission.
  A. Transfusion of blood products (Figure 8-5). Highest incidence of the disease is in those receiving 1, 2, or 4 listed here.
    1. Whole blood.
    2. Red blood cells.
    3. Fresh frozen plasma.
    4. Deglycerolized RBCs.
    5. Platelet concentrate.
  B. Needle stick or puncture wound from a blood-contaminated item.
  C. Nonpercutaneous spread similar to hepatitis B (suspected, not proven).

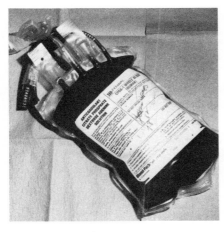

Figure 8-5: Blood for transfusion is the primary source of non-A, non-B hepatitis infection.

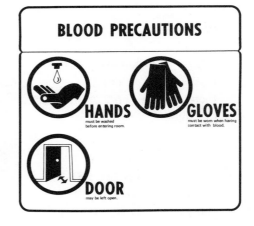

Figure 8-6: Blood precautions are used in cases of non-A, non-B hepatitis infection. (Courtesy, St. Joseph's Hospital, Tampa.)

IV. Clinical picture.
  A. Incubation period of 14 to 115 days (mean 50 days).
  B. Clinical course.
    1. Similar to hepatitis B, but not as severe.
    2. About two-thirds of cases are anicteric.
    3. Progresses to chronic active hepatitis more often than does hepatitis B.

V. Isolation and precautions.
  A. Blood precautions (Figure 8-6).
    1. Wear gloves whenever handling blood or secretion- or excretion-contaminated items.
    2. Use an impervious puncture-resistant container for all needles and sharp instruments.
      a.) Do not recap needles.
      b.) Do not bend or break needles.
    3. Label laboratory specimens "Hepatitis."
  B. Proper cleanup of blood spills.
    1. Wipe up spill with a disposable cloth.
    2. Flood area with disinfectant active against hepatitis B.
    3. Wipe up with a disposable cloth.
    4. Discard rags in a bag.
    5. Seal and discard bag.
  C. Wear gloves when handling blood or body excretions or secretions from any patient, since the patient may have asymptomatic hepatitis. Patients with a history of receiving blood products pose the greatest risk to hospital employees.

VI. Patient teaching.
  A. Instruct patient in use of individual personal-care items, procedures, and practices.
    1. There must be no sharing of razors, styptic pencils, toothbrushes, towels, and the like.
    2. Female patients should bag sanitary napkins in plastic bags and use care in choosing a place to discard them.
    3. Patients should be instructed not to pick at blemishes, cuts, scratches, and to keep any open lesions covered.
    4. Proper hand washing is important, especially after activities in which blood contamination is possible.

B. Family should be instructed that only risk of acquiring disease is from entry of infected blood into their bodies.

VII. Prophylaxis.
   A. There should first be documented exposure to an infected patient.
      1. Infected blood enters an existing open wound, scratch, or the like.
      2. Infected blood contacts a mucous membrane surface, such as an eye, the mouth, nose.
      3. A cut, scratch, or wound occurs with an item contaminated with infected blood.
   B. Immune serum globulin 0.06 ml/kg immediately and repeated in 30 days.

VIII. Prevention.
   A. Use care in handling all blood products.
      1. Blood products administered to patients.
      2. Blood specimens from patients.
      3. Any blood spill.
      4. Control serum in laboratory.
   B. Utilize safety precautions when caring for patients.
      1. Wear gloves whenever performing a venipuncture.
      2. Place infected patients on blood precautions.
      3. Note in patient record any drug abuse history or history of receiving blood products in the last six months.
         a.) Observe for possible disease.
         b.) Alert other personnel of record notation.

T·E·S·T

Hepatitis A

1. True/False
   A. ____ Patients infected with hepatitis A need not be isolated in the hospital if they are educable, cooperative, and not fecally incontinent.
   B. ____ Most hepatitis A infections are caused by exposure to infected blood.
   C. ____ Hepatitis A has an abrupt onset and always is symptomatic.
   D. ____ Ambulatory patients diagnosed with hepatitis A should be discouraged from using public eating and restroom facilities in the hospital.
   E. ____ The severity of hepatitis A increases with age.
2. List five symptoms of hepatitis A.

Answers are on page 230.

A·N·S·W·E·R·S

Hepatitis A

1. True/False
   A. False. Patients in the preicteric phase and during the first week of icterus have, in addition to infectious stool, other body secretions that may be infectious. For that reason, enteric precautions are used during that period.
   B. False. Hepatitis A infections are almost always acquired by exposure to virus-containing body excretions or food or water contaminated with these excretions. The period of blood viremia in hepatitis A is very brief; therefore, blood transmission is rare.
   C. False. Hepatitis A most often has an abrupt onset but it may be insidious. The vast majority of patients with hepatitis A have no recognizable symptoms.
   D. True. Such patients may inadvertently contaminate items in these facilities.
   E. True. Hepatitis A in young infants is usually asymptomatic and in children is generally a mild disease. In adults, hepatitis frequently requires bed rest and/or hospitalization.
2. Loss of appetite, loss of taste for cigarettes, itching, nausea and vomiting, aching joints, fever, weakness, and mild abdominal pain and tenderness.

T·E·S·T

Hepatitis B

1. True/False
   A. _____ Five to 10 percent of persons with a history of hepatitis B are carriers.
   B. _____ All body excretions/secretions of a patient with hepatitis B are infectious.
   C. _____ Antibody to hepatitis B always persists lifelong.
   D. _____ Hepatitis B may be anicteric and asymptomatic.
   E. _____ Hepatitis B may have a sexual mode of spread.
2. List five symptoms of hepatitis B.
3. A patient (cooperative and educable) diagnosed as having hepatitis B should be placed on
   a. blood precautions.   b. enteric precautions.
   c. excretion precautions.   d. strict isolation.
4. The hospitalized patient on precautions for hepatitis B may
   a. walk in the hall.
   b. use public restrooms in the hospital.
   c. use public eating facilities in the hospital.
5. Patient teaching should include
   a. instructions in basic hand washing and hygiene.
   b. how to care for soiled clothing.
   c. how to care for dishware.
   d. how to decontaminate his toilet facility.
6. Personnel exposed to HBV should
   a. always be given anti-HBs.
   b. be evaluated as to type of exposure and given the appropriate globulin.
   c. have the globulin repeated in 30 days.
7. Key safety imperatives employees should be aware of to prevent acquisition of hepatitis B include
   a. always wear gloves when working with blood products.
   b. place all needles and sharp objects in impervious containers.
   c. never break needles or syringes.
   d. all the above.

Answers are on page 232.

231

A·N·S·W·E·R·S

Hepatitis B

1. True/False
   A. True. Overall, one percent of the general population carries hepatitis B, and five to 10 percent of those with recognized illness go on to the carrier state.
   B. False. The stool of individuals with hepatitis B contains some material that neutralizes hepatitis B virus. Therefore, unless it is grossly contaminated with blood, stool is not infectious.
   C. False. In a small proportion of patients, antibody to hepatitis B becomes undetectable after various periods of convalescence.
   D. True. In certain categories of patients, such as dialysis patients, asymptomatic disease is the rule rather than the exception. Overall, at least 50 percent of patients with hepatitis B have no symptoms or jaundice.
   E. True. Hepatitis B is spread between husbands and wives as well as among male homosexuals. The precise mechanism of sexual spread, however, is not clearly defined.
2. Itching, skin rash, nausea, loss of appetite, loss of taste for cigarettes, joint pains, muscle aching, fever, weakness.
3. a. blood precautions.
4. a. walk in the hall.
5. a. instructions in basic hand washing and hygiene.
   b. how to care for soiled clothing.
6. b. be evaluated as to type of exposure and given the appropriate globulin.
   c. should have the globulin repeated in 30 days.
7. d. all above answers, a–c.

T·E·S·T

Non-A, non-B
hepatitis

1. True/False. Non-A, non-B hepatitis represents 80 to 90 percent of all transfusion-associated hepatitis.
2. List the three blood products that have the highest occurrence of non-A, non-B hepatitis.
3. Describe the three occurrences that represent exposure to non-A, non-B hepatitis (exposure to patient or patient's blood).

Answers are on page 234.

A·N·S·W·E·R·S

Non-A, non-B hepatitis

1. True. Since blood donated for transfusion in the United States is now routinely screened for hepatitis B, the incidence of transfusion-associated hepatitis B has fallen dramatically, leaving non-A, non-B hepatitis as the dominant transfusion-associated infection.
2. Whole blood, packed red blood cells, and deglycerolized red blood cells.
3. A. Infected blood enters an existing open wound, scratch, or the like.
   B. Infected blood contacts a mucous membrane surface.
   C. An item contaminated with infected blood causes a cut, scratch, or wound.

9

Meningitis

Purpose

Meningitis, an inflammatory disease of the central nervous system, is a medical emergency requiring early diagnosis and rapid initiation of rational therapy. Although meningitis may be the sequela of a variety of irritating substances introduced into the meninges, such as chemical agents, or the result of trauma or tumor, the purpose of this section is to understand the viral, bacterial, and fungal causes of meningitis.

Meningeal manifestations of CNS infections may be aseptic (lymphocytic) or suppurative (PMNs). Meningitis is the result of direct invasion of organisms and/or a hematogenous dissemination of organisms from an antecedent infection. In adults and older children, hematogenous spread can occur from remote foci, such as the lungs, intestines, skin, paranasal sinus, or from neuroorthopedic infections (as a result of congenital neuromalformations or procedures) or trauma.

Fetal and neonatal infections occur hematogenously from the pharynx or GI tract as a result of aspiration of contaminated amniotic fluid, colonization in utero, or during passage through the birth canal. Additional potential sources of infection for neonates include personnel, life support systems, and contaminated equipment.

Other factors that influence susceptibility are immunosuppression, chronic underlying illness (sickle cell disease, alcoholism, and leukemia), and age (prematurity or advanced age).

Meningitis

Learning objectives

○ Know routes of transmission of bacterial, viral, and fungal meningitis.

○ List the most common causative agents.

○ Recognize various clinical presentations.

○ Identify predisposing factors and methods of prevention.

Behavioral objectives

○ Promptly identify suspect patients.

○ Communicate information about isolation protocol to employees, patients, and visitors.

I. Bacterial meningitis: Bacterial meningitis is a suppurative form of meningeal reaction. Central nervous system (CNS) infections can occur as a result of primary (direct) or secondary (metastatic) invasion by the organism. Primary invasion occurs in the absence of an antecedent infection and the portal of entry may be clinically inapparent. Secondary invasion occurs as the result of an antecedent infection via hematogenous dissemination of the organism. Certain individuals, because of a chronic underlying disease (sickle cell disease, alcoholism, leukemia, or lymphoma) or age (premature infants and elderly) are at greater risk. Often signs and symptoms are obscure in the compromised host.

A. *Neisseria meningitidis* (cerebrospinal fever, epidemic meningitis, meningococcal infection, meningococcemia, and spotted fever).

1. Epidemiology.

a.) Epidemic—usually associated with crowded living quarters such as military barracks, camps, institutions, and schools.

b.) Increased incidence during winter.

c.) May occur at any age, but generally more prevalent among infants and children.

d.) Occurs among males more than females.

e.) Onset of disease related to fatigue and overcrowding.

f.) Four serogroups A, B, C, Y.

2. Transmission.

a.) Droplet or direct contact with nasal and throat discharges from infected individuals.

b.) Asymptomatic carriers may serve as reservoirs of infection.

c.) Most infections prior to initiation of therapy.

d.) Man is the only reservoir.

3. Incubation period: two to 10 days, with three to four days most common.

4. Signs and symptoms: The three phases of meningococcal diseases and associated signs and symptoms are as follows:

    a.) Phase I: Local or nasopharyngeal infection (colonization).

        (1.) Often asymptomatic or with mild URI.

        (2.) Recognized only in cultures.

        (3.) Source of infection to others.

    b.) Phase II: Septicemia (meningococcemia with or without meningitis).

        (1.) Petechiae appear.

        (2.) The skin lesions are usually generalized in infants.

        (3.) In children and adults, lesions are most often on the legs.

        (4.) Early in the illness, a morbilliform rash, resembling measles, appears on trunk and lower extremities.

        (5.) Progresses from rash to petechia within hours.

        (6.) In petechial stage, characteristics range from minute to large and may appear ecchymotic or purpuric.

        (7.) May be associated with fulminant course.

    c.) Phase III: Clinical evidence of meningitis.

        (1.) Characteristic signs and symptoms appear: stiff neck, headache (severe, throbbing), fever, chills, backache, and vomiting.

        (2.) Death may occur within four hours of onset.

5. Prevention.

    a.) Maintain good personal hygiene.

    b.) Avoid direct contact or droplet contact of infected persons.

    c.) Keep in respiratory isolation until 24 hours after effective therapy has begun.

6. Prophylaxis: rifampin or minocycline.
   a.) For household members.
   b.) For hospital employees having prolonged intimate contact without maintaining proper precautions.

B. *Haemophilus influenzae.*
   1. Epidemiology.
      a.) Six antigenic types identified.
      b.) Virulence apparently linked to type of antigen, with type B most common.
      c.) Infants six months to three years most susceptible because they lack protective antibody.
      d.) Associated with carrier state.
      e.) May or may not cause clinical symptoms.
      f.) May begin as URI and progress to bacteremia and/or meningitis.
   2. Transmission.
      a.) Person-to-person.
      b.) Occurs rapidly and extensively in nurseries.
   3. Prevention: no isolation (respiratory isolation in nursery).
   4. Signs and symptoms.
      a.) Associated with carrier state with or without clinical illness.
      b.) Clinical illness may present as URI, such as epiglottitis or otitis media, or as LRI (pneumonia).
      c.) May progress to bacteremia and meningitis.
      d.) Fever, sore throat, hoarseness, barking cough.
      e.) May progress to fulminant course within hours.

C. *Streptococcus pneumoniae* (pneumococcus).
   1. Epidemiology—occurs most often in
      a.) Infants with otitis media, mastoiditis, pneumonia.
      b.) Elderly—associated with pneumonia and alcoholism.
      c.) Other age groups—associated with skull fractures.
      d.) Sickle cell disease a predisposing factor at any age.
      e.) Associated with carrier state.
   2. Transmission: direct contact or infected droplets.
   3. Prevention/control: no isolation.
   4. Prophylaxis: none.

D. *Escherichia coli.*

1. Most common cause of neonatal meningitis. It is thought that invasive properties of the organism and neonatal infection are linked to *E. coli* strains with a K_1 capsular antigen.

2. Colonization and resultant infection of neonates occurs during passage through the birth canal and/or from nursery personnel who may be carriers.

3. Transmission: person-to-person, usually via hands and contaminated equipment.

4. Isolation: neonates in incubator for 24 hours to 48 hours until organism identified.

E. *Streptococcus pyogenes* (groups A and B).

1. Can usually be found in the respiratory, GI, and genital tracts.

2. Fetal infection can occur as the result of aspiration of contaminated amniotic fluid; infection in the neonate may result from colonization during passage through the birth canal.

3. In older children and adults, it is usually due to antecedent infection of lung, intestine, skin, paranasal sinus, ENT, or because of infection resulting from trauma or neuroorthopedic procedures.

F. *Staphylococcus aureus.*

1. Part of the normal skin and nasal flora.

2. Meningitis may occur as the result of antecedent infection of the skin or paranasal sinus or infection due to trauma, congenital neuromalformations, or neuroorthopedic procedures.

3. Transmission: from individuals with staphylococcus infections or from nasal carriers. Most common route is via hands.

4. Isolation: none, unless there is frank wound or respiratory infection.

G. *Klebsiella pneumoniae, Salmonella, Pseudomonas, Listeria monocytogenes.*

1. *Klebsiella pneumoniae*—part of the fecal flora of humans and animals. Common in neurosurgery infections.

2. *Salmonella*—rarely a cause of meningitis. Natural reservoir—wild and domestic animals.

   3. *Pseudomonas*—a common cause of traumatic or
      neurosurgery infections.
   4. *Listeria monocytogenes*—easily mistaken for diphtheroids.
      Most often infects neonates and immune-suppressed
      patients.
   5. Isolation: none.
H. *Mycobacterium tuberculosis.*
   1. Only reservoir is man.
   2. Spreads via airborne droplets from open lung infections.
   3. Reaches meninges by hematogenous spread from lung or
      other extraneural focus.
   4. Clinically may mimic viral or fungal meningitis.
   5. Requires isolation only when associated with active lung
      infection.

II. Viral meningitis.
   A. Enteroviruses, including poliovirus, coxsackievirus, and
      echovirus: Natural host for enteroviruses is man. These viruses
      are transmitted from person to person either by direct contact
      with infected feces (fecal-oral route), by ingestion of virus-
      contaminated water or milk, or via respiratory secretions. They
      are excreted in feces, and when large numbers accumulate in
      sewage there is danger of contamination of water in wells,
      pools, and streams, in addition to drinking-water supplies.
      Because infection in young children may be mild or
      asymptomatic, day-care centers have become foci of spread in
      communities. Secretion precautions or enteric precautions for
      infected patients are generally suggested.
   B. Mumps virus: Man is the natural host for mumps virus. This
      virus is transmitted through direct contact with infected saliva
      or droplet nuclei or by fomites that have been freshly
      contaminated. Respiratory precautions are used. Invasion of
      the CNS is a frequent complication of mumps; however, its
      sequelae may vary from asymptomatic to a mild meningeal
      irritation to a more severe encephalitis.
   C. Lymphocytic choriomeningitis (LCM): Animals, especially
      mice, are the natural hosts for this virus. Pet hamsters, guinea
      pigs, dogs, monkeys, and swine have also been implicated in
      the transmission of the disease. The virus is excreted in saliva,
      urine, feces, and semen of the infected animal. Transmission
      to man occurs via contaminated food or dust. This disease has

a wide spectrum of clinical manifestations ranging from flu-like symptoms to hemorrhagic meningoencephalitis. The latter occurs rarely in men. Isolation is not practiced, since diagnosis is delayed and person-to-person transmission rare.

   D. Herpesvirus hominis type II: This is a common cause of sexually transmitted genital infection. In women, and to a lesser extent in men, primary genital herpes frequently ascends the nerve roots or travels the bloodstream to cause a self-limited aseptic meningitis. Recurrences may accompany cutaneous exacerbation. Other viruses associated with meningitis are zoster, measles, hepatitis, adenoviruses, and rhinovirus.

III. Fungal meningitis.
   A. *Cryptococcus neoformans* is a fungus found in pigeon droppings, where it replicates and may remain viable for up to two years. It is transmitted to man through inhalation of dust contaminated with the live fungus. The immunosuppressed (oncology) and the high-risk patients (alcoholics, diabetics) are more prone to develop the disease. However, many individuals with no underlying problems are found to have cryptococcosis. This disease may vary from a mild pulmonary illness to meningitis and indeed has a predilection for the central nervous system.
   B. *Coccidioides immitis,* a fungus that causes valley fever, is found in the arid and semiarid soil of the Southwestern U.S., Mexico, and South America. Transmission to man occurs through inhalation of dust or soil contaminated with the fungus. Disease in the lungs may vary from localized pneumonitis to chronic cavity disease that resembles tuberculosis. Dissemination from the lungs may reach any tissue of the body, and the leptomeninges are frequently involved.
   C. *Histoplasma capsulatum* is a fungus that in tissue grows as a yeast but on laboratory medium grows as a mold. It is found in the droppings of birds, such as chickens, blackbirds, and starlings, and of bats. Again, transmission to man occurs through inhalation of contaminated dust or soil particles. Disease in the lung may vary from acute benign respiratory illness to chronic pulmonary disease resembling tuberculosis. When dissemination occurs, the CNS is a vulnerable target.
   D. *Blastomyces dermatitidis* is a yeast of unknown source in nature. Common infection is in skin, bone, and lung;

meningitis is rare. Person-to-person transmission occurs only by direct contact. Use skin and wound precautions for skin lesions.

E. *Candida species* are rare causes of meningitis, most often occurring in diabetics and cancer patients. Since *Candida* are part of normal upper respiratory flora, isolation is not used.

IV. Protozoa.

A. *Toxoplasma gondii* is a common cause of protozoan human infection. It occurs in feline feces and raw meat. Meningitis may occur in the immune-deficient host. Isolation is not used.

B. *Naeglaria* and *Acanthamoeba,* fresh water amebae, are rare causes of human meningitis. The disease comes from swimming in contaminated fresh water, is not communicated person-to-person, and is almost always fatal.

V. Generalizations about meningitis.

A. Host susceptibility and pathogenesis.

1. Most episodes occur in normal hosts.

2. Certain uncommon organisms cause meningitis in immune-compromised hosts. These include listeria, mycobacteria, fungi, and parasites.

3. Access to the meninges may be through direct inoculation, blood-borne spread, or along nerve fibers. Direct inoculation can occur with trauma or neurosurgical procedures. Soil organisms and nosocomial bacteria predominate. Hematogenous spread is the most common; pneumococci, *Haemophilus influenzae,* and meningococci are the most common organisms in this class. Viruses such as poliovirus and herpesvirus may enter along peripheral nerves, coxsackievirus and herpesvirus may also invade via the bloodstream.

4. Repeated episodes of bacterial meningitis should suggest an anatomic defect in the neural coverings, such as fractured cribriform plate or petrous ridge or congenital defect. Certain organisms may specifically invade neural tissue because of surface organelles, which cause them to adhere to nerve cells or adjacent tissues.

B. Symptoms.

1. Symptoms are determined by both the invading organism and the underlying state of the host.

2. Adults with bacterial meningitis have rigors, fever, malaise, and stiff neck with headache.

3. Infants with bacterial meningitis have stupor, coma, flaccidity, and fever with or without stiff neck.

4. Vomiting, dizziness, seizures, and delirium are common at all ages.

5. Patients with viral meningitis have diarrhea, myalgia, pharyngitis, cough, photophobia, retroorbital pain, fever, headache, stiff neck.

C. Clinical, laboratory, and X-ray findings.

1. See above for common clinical symptoms.

2. Increased pressure within the skull may cause bulging of the fontanelles in infants and blurring of margins of the optic nerve in the retina at all ages.

3. Fungal and tuberculous meningitis are most often chronic and may mimic tumors.

4. Laboratory findings.

    a.) CBC—high WBC with bacterial meningitis, normal or low in other forms.

    b.) Urinalysis—high urine concentration is the most common abnormality.

    c.) Other tests.

        (1.) CSF cell differential shows mostly PMNs with bacterial, lymphocytes with viral, meningitis.

        (2.) Sugar generally low with TB and with bacterial or fungal meningitis; it may be slightly low with viral meningitis, but it is generally normal.

        (3.) Protein is markedly elevated with bacterial, moderately with viral, meningitis.

        (4.) Cultures of spinal fluid should be done for bacteria, fungi, and mycobacteria.

        (5.) If available, virus cultures should be used as well as acute and convalescent serum antibody titers.

        (6.) Gram stain is important, but requires expert interpretation.

D. Differential diagnosis.

1. Tumor.

2. Leukemia.

3. Vasculitis.

         4. Infectious endocarditis.

         5. Infected parameningeal focus.

E. Prognosis.

    1. Complications—cranial nerve palsies, blindness, deafness, motor or intellectual defects, hydrocephalus, abscess, subdural effusion, death.

    2. Death from untreated disease occurs in 100 percent of patients with bacterial meningitis, less than 10 percent of those with viral meningitis. Chronic meningitis causes death in about 80 percent of untreated patients. Treatment reduces mortality from bacterial meningitis to five to 35 percent, in chronic meningitis to approximately 20 to 30 percent, but has little effect on mortality of viral meningitis.

F. Medical treatment.

    1. Goals are to sterilize the infection foci and to prevent sequelae of inflammation.

    2. Not all antibiotics enter the spinal fluid well from the bloodstream. Therefore, selection of treatment regimen is a challenging clinical test.

    3. Certain antimicrobials need to be injected directly into the spinal fluid for maximum effectiveness.

    4. Steroids may be helpful in reducing inflammation and results of inflammation.

    5. Fluids may be restricted to reduce brain edema.

T·E·S·T

1. Meningitis is
   a. inflammation of the linings of the brain and spinal cord.
   b. always fatal.
   c. always highly contagious.
   d. caused only by bacteria.

2. Meningitis may be caused by
   a. bacteria.
   b. viruses.
   c. fungi.
   d. protozoa.
   e. tumors.
   f. all of the above.

3. Isolation for meningitis
   a. is always strict.
   b. is never necessary.
   c. depends on the suspected cause.

4. If the entity is common in bacterial meningitis, mark "A"; if in viral, mark "B."
   _____ CSF very high in PMNs.
   _____ low sugar.
   _____ fecal-oral transmission.
   _____ CSF very high in lymphocytes.

5. Organisms reach the meninges by
   a. hematogenous spread.
   b. lymphatics.
   c. spread along peripheral nerves.
   d. direct inoculation.
   e. contiguous spread from adjacent foci.
   f. all of the above.

6. The clinical hallmarks of meningitis are
   a. confusion.
   b. fever.
   c. stiff neck.
   d. seizures.
   e. all of the above.

Test continued on next page.

7. If Strict Isolation indicated, mark "SI"; if wound and skin, "W & S"; if respiratory, "RI"; if enteric, "EI"; if none, "NI."
   _____ Meningococcal meningitis.
   _____ *Haemophilus influenzae* meningitis.
   _____ Pneumococcal meningitis.
   _____ TB meningitis (normal chest X-ray).
   _____ TB meningitis (cavities on chest X-ray).
   _____ Enteroviral meningitis.

A·N·S·W·E·R·S

1. a. inflammation of the linings of the brain and spinal cord.
2. f. all of the answers, a–e.
3. c. depends on the suspected cause.
4. A CSF very high in PMNs.
   A low sugar.
   B fecal-oral transmission.
   B CSF very high in lymphocytes.
5. f. all of the answers, a–e.
6. e. all of the answers, a–d.
7. RI Meningococcal meningitis.
   NI *Haemophilus influenzae* meningitis (RI in nursery).
   NI Pneumococcal meningitis.
   NI TB meningitis (normal chest X-ray).
   RI TB meningitis (cavities on chest X-ray).
   EI Enteroviral meningitis.

10

Scabies and pediculosis

Purpose

This section deals with the infectious diseases caused by mites and lice. The goal is to understand the epidemiological characteristics of the diseases and how to prevent their spread.

Learning objectives

o State clinical signs of disease, living habits of mites and lice.

o List and define identification methods.

o Describe isolation procedures and treatment techniques.

o Explain community prevention, including the steps in the education of the patient and family to prevent the spread of the disease to others.

Behavioral objectives

o Conduct efficient examinations for infestation.

o Treat patients effectively.

o Provide helpful patient instruction.

Scabies

Scabies is considered an infectious disease of the skin. It is characterized by visible papules or vesicles with linear burrows containing the mites and their eggs.

I. Causative organism—mite known as *Sarcoptes scabiei* (Figure 10-1).
   A. Female mite.
      1. Oval shape, flat vertically and curved dorsally, 0.4 × 0.3 mm in size. Four pairs of legs, two posterior and two anterior.
      2. Moves moderately rapidly on surface of skin, one inch per minute.
      3. Lives in burrows in superficial layers of skin.

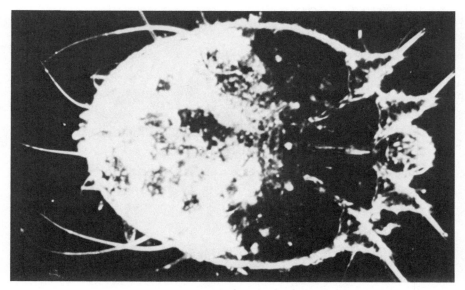

Figure 10-1: *Sarcoptes scabiei*. (Reproduced with permission of Reed and Carnrick.)

B. Male mite.
1. Size is 0.2 × 1.5 mm.
2. Adult usually lives on the skin but may dig a burrow for food. He may also enter the burrow of a female to mate.

II. Epidemiology.
   A. It is seldom seen with good hygiene, being especially common in armies, prisons, and in areas of poverty.
   B. Usually contracted through contact with infected individuals. Rarely are clothing, bed linens, or towels the source, even if contaminated with the adult female or its eggs, larvae, or nymphs. Organisms may survive in linens for brief time.
   C. May be spread by sexual contact. Scabies in young adults may signify promiscuous sexuality. Look for other sexually transmitted diseases.

III. Pathogenesis.
   A. The fertilized female lays eggs in burrows. She lives four to five weeks and lays one to two eggs daily.
   B. Eggs hatch in three to five days.
   C. The newly hatched larvae either stay in the burrow or migrate to the skin surface and cling to the base of the hair follicles. Here they pass through two nymph stages.
   D. Eight to 16 days after the eggs are laid, the young become adults. The cycle begins again as the female begins laying eggs.
   E. Initially, there is little or no itching or rash. As allergy to the mites develops (about four to six weeks), an itchy rash appears. Re-exposure has shorter incubation period.
   F. Clinical illness may last one to two months.

IV. Infection manifestations.
   A. Burrows usually found in the spaces between fingers, backs of hands, elbows, armpits, groin, abdomen. Face is not involved in adults, but may be in children. The burrow usually consists of a short, wavy, dirty appearing line. At the distal end is a tiny blister.
   B. Intense itching in early morning hours may keep the infected person awake.

Scabies and pediculosis

    C. Scratching makes the area red and excoriated. Secondary bacterial infection often occurs.

V. Diagnosis.
    A. Equipment: strong light, magnifying glass, sterile needle (hypodermic or IV), glass slide.
    B. Mite can usually be found in the blister or burrow.

VI. Clinical forms of scabies.
    A. In clean individuals (cleanliness not totally preventive).
       1. Findings minimal.
       2. Burrows hard to find.
    B. Incognito
       1. Mistakenly treated with corticosteroids that mask signs and symptoms.
       2. Infestation not cured, transmissibility not altered.
       3. Simulates a variety of other situations.
    C. Nodular.
       1. Occurs on covered areas of the body, most commonly groin, axillary region, and male genitalia.
       2. Reddish-brown pruritic nodules may persist from months to more than a year, despite repeated therapy.
       3. Exaggerated hypersensitivity disappears spontaneously.
    D. Infants and young children.
       1. Usually lack burrows.
       2. Skin changes nonspecific.
       3. Atypical distribution: head, neck, palms, and soles of the feet.
       4. Secondary skin infections.
       5. Bullae and vesicles may occur.
    E. Crusted (Norwegian) scabies.
       1. Rare disease.
       2. Highly contagious, even on casual contact, because of the vast number of mites in the scales and the length of time before diagnosis.
       3. Predilection for mentally retarded, physically and immunologically debilitated.
       4. Seldom occurs in normal healthy individuals.

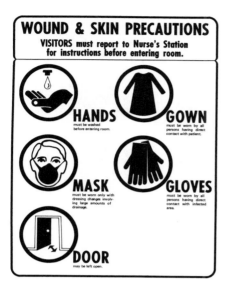

WOUND & SKIN PRECAUTIONS
VISITORS must report to Nurse's Station
for instructions before entering room.

HANDS
must be washed
before entering room.

GOWN
must be worn by all
persons having direct
contact with patient.

MASK
must be worn only with
dressing changes involv-
ing large amounts of
drainage.

GLOVES
must be worn by all
persons having direct
contact with infected
area.

DOOR
may be left open.

Figure 10-2: Wound and skin precautions are used for patients with scabies. (Courtesy, St. Joseph's Hospital, Tampa.)

VII. Prevention.

    A. Isolation of the patient.

        1. Wound and skin precautions (Figure 10-2) maintained for 24 hours after treatment began.

        2. A second treatment in a week is to make certain all eggs are destroyed.

    B. Isolation of personnel.

        1. Personnel diagnosed as having scabies should remain off-duty for 24 hours after treatment is completed.

        2. Other personnel exposed to an infected person should not be treated routinely, but should be observed for symptoms. Prolonged close contact may justify prophylaxis.

        3. A second treatment is optional a week after the first, to be certain all the eggs are destroyed.

VIII. Medications.

    A. Lindane (gamma benzene hexachloride) (Kwell).

    B. Crotamiton (Eurax).

    C. Precipitated sulfur (Liquimat, Meted).

    D. Pyrethrins (A-200 Pyrinate, R&C Spray).

Scabies and pediculosis

IX. Treatment procedure.
   A. Doctor's order necessary.
   B. Follow the directions on the medication, especially in pregnancy.
   C. Treat all bed partners or family members.
   D. With reinfection, an antihistamine may be added for four or five days.
   E. The above procedures also apply to personnel who inadvertently become infected through patient contact.

X. Home instructions.
   A. Avoid direct skin contact with infected areas.
   B. Avoid contact with soiled linen.
   C. Use all fresh linens. This includes clothing, towels, and bed linens.
   D. Soiled clothing and linens are cared for as in wound and skin precautions.
   E. Avoid sharing hand-drying materials used by others.
   F. Linens are to be washed in hot soapy water and dried thoroughly.
   G. Anything that cannot be washed should be dry-cleaned if possible. Storage of items that cannot be cleaned for 10 days or more may reduce infectivity.
   H. If mattress is not plastic-covered, enclose in air-tight plastic bag for 10 days. May be sprayed with gamma benzene hexachloride before enclosing.

Pediculosis

Pediculosis is a general term applied to infestation of the skin with lice. It is associated with intense itching and rash.

I. Causative organisms.
   A. Crab louse (*Phthirus pubis*).
   B. Head louse (*Pediculus capitis*, Figure 10-3).
   C. Body louse (*Pediculus corporis*).
   D. Lice are small, flat, wingless insects with stubby antennae and three pairs of legs that end in sharp, curved claws. Head, body, and pubic lice pass through similar life cycles, developing from eggs that take about a week to incubate.
   E. The eggs (nits) of pubic and head lice are tear-shaped and are found on the shafts of the hairs close to the body.

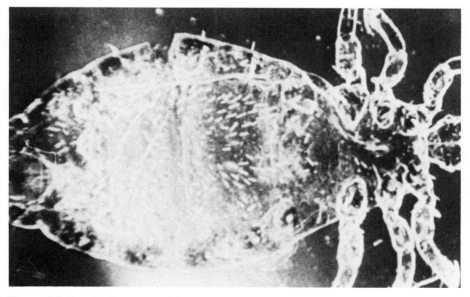

Figure 10-3: *Pediculus capitis.*
(*Reproduced with permission of Reed and Carnrick.*)

253

Scabies and pediculosis

II. Epidemiology.
   A. Lice can spread despite a high general level of cleanliness.
   B. Infection with body or pubic lice usually occurs with intimate contact (sleeping in the same bed or wearing the infested person's clothes).
   C. Head lice are acquired through using the infested person's comb or wearing his hat.
   D. Upholstered furniture and bedding also may be potential reservoirs.
   E. Body lice transmit epidemic typhus, trench fever, and a louse-borne variety of relapsing fever (Borrelia).
   F. Body lice are rather rare in the United States.
   G. Head and pubic lice are not directly implicated in disease transmission.
   H. Head lice tend to infect schoolchildren. Pubic lice tend to infect young adults. Body lice can be found in any age group. Lice from lower animals do not infest man.

III. Pathogenesis.
   A. Body lice deposit their eggs upon fibers of clothing, particularly seams.
   B. The immature nymphs become mature in about three weeks.
   C. Each mature louse survives about a month. During this time, the female can produce five to 10 eggs per day and as many as 300 in her lifetime.
   D. Head and pubic lice are highly dependent on humans for daily blood meals and warmth of the body. They will die if separated from the host for 24 hours.
   E. The body louse can live in clothing and survive up to a week without a human blood meal.

IV. Signs, symptoms, and diagnosis: Several weeks may elapse between infestation and occurrence of signs or symptoms. Maturation of nymphs takes a week and only then do they begin to lay eggs. It will be another week before these hatch. (It takes a while to build up enough of a "flock" to see.) Itching does not occur until the patient develops hypersensitivity.
   A. Equipment: strong light, magnifying glass, fine-tooth comb, glass slide.
   B. Pediculosis capitis: Pruritus is a cardinal symptom, though not always present. Diagnosis is most often made by identifying

the nits cemented to the hair at the hair-skin junction. Comb hair with a very-fine-tooth comb over a dark surface or onto a glass slide. Remove one of the hairs and examine under the microscope or with a magnifying glass. Pyoderma and regional adenopathy may be a result of the severe scratching and secondary infection.

C. Pediculosis corporis: Numerous excoriations due to the severe itching will be found on the trunk and neck. Bacterial infection is a common complication. The lice will be found crawling on the seams of clothing and in the armpits, beltline, and collar while they feed on the host.

D. Pediculosis pubis: The diagnosis is usually made by the scratching and the presence of nits on the pubic hair. It is not an epidemic disease, being spread by intimate body contact and less often through clothing and bedding. The lice may also be found on other hairy portions of the lower abdomen, thighs, and buttocks.

E. Affected skin may appear brown. As the lice feed they defecate, and one can see the brownish stain of excrement.

V. Methods of treatment.
   A. Until the 19th century, the only treatments were absolute body cleanliness, frequent change of clothing, and shaving of the head.
   B. Early in the 20th century, mercuric ointment, copper, crude oil, and kerosene were found effective. The treatments took several days and were often dangerous.
   C. New usage of pesticides, such as DDT, has been very effective. Use of them made WW II the first war that was not followed by a typhus epidemic, although typhus was prevalent in the Italian campaign.
   D. Since the ban on DDT new products are being sought.
   E. The products being used are lindane (gamma benzene hexachloride) (Kwell), pyrethrin (RID Pediculicide), and malathion lotion 0.5 percent. This last is not frequently used in the U.S.
   F. Treatment techniques.
      1. Use the shampoo or treatment ordered following the manufacturer's suggestions.
      2. Clean all personal articles at time of treatment, such as combs, brushes, and clothing. Wash in hot (130°F) soapy

water, or dry-clean. Clean beds, vacuuming all seams to remove dust, and spray with a pyrethrin spray.

3. Repeat in one week if clinical symptoms continue, to be sure all eggs are destroyed.

VI. Prevention and isolation.
   A. Family.
      1. Inspect all family members at time of diagnosis and for two weeks afterward. Treat if any persons are infested.
      2. Good personal hygiene and daily clothing changes are useful.
      3. Advise not to use anyone else's personal items or wear their clothing.
      4. Warn that reinfestation can occur.
   B. Notify local health department if the patient is a school-aged child. There may be an epidemic in the school system.
   C. Isolation.
      1. As soon as diagnosed and until 24 hours after the application of the pediculicide.
      2. The patient is placed on wound and skin precautions.
      3. Infested hospital personnel must remain off-duty until the pediculicide has been in contact with the affected area for at least 24 hours.

T·E·S·T

1. Scabies is an infectious disease.
   a. of childhood only.
   b. of the skin.
   c. of rural areas only.
   d. all of the above.
2. Scabies is caused by
   a. mites.
   b. bacteria.
   c. protozoa.
   d. none of the above.
3. The mite digs its burrows
   a. between the fingers.

    b. in the axilla.

    c. in the groin.

    d. all of the above.

4. The isolation precautions to use are

    a. protective.

    b. enteric.

    c. wound and skin.

    d. strict.

5. Treatment is

    a. done once and repeated in a week.

    b. left on the skin for 24 hours.

    c. done after a warm shower or bath.

    d. all of the above.

6. Pediculosis affects

    a. young children.

    b. teens and young adults.

    c. adults.

    d. all of the above.

7. Pediculosis is caused by

    a. head lice.

    b. body lice.

    c. pubic lice.

    d. all of the above.

8. The items most helpful in making a diagnosis of pediculosis are

    a. a strong light.

    b. a light surface.

    c. a very-fine-tooth comb.

    d. needle.

9. The isolation precaution to use in pediculosis is

    a. strict for 48 hours.

    b. wound and skin for 24 hours.

    c. enteric for 36 hours.

    d. protective for 48 hours.

Answers are on page 258.

A·N·S·W·E·R·S

1. b. of the skin.
2. a. mites.
3. d. all of the answers, a–c.
4. c. wound and skin.
5. d. all of the answers, a–c.
6. d. all of the answers, a–c.
7. d. all of the answers, a–c.
8. a. a strong light.
   c. a very-fine-tooth comb.
9. b. wound and skin for 24 hours.

11

Tuberculosis

Purpose

Tuberculosis is a disease with which most health-care personnel are familiar. This section is designed to correct any misconceptions concerning cause, transmission, and cure of the disease.

Learning objectives

○ List routes of transmission of tuberculosis.

○ Know the frequency of the disease.

○ Identify various clinical presentations of tuberculosis.

○ Describe techniques to restrict spread of the disease.

Behavioral objectives

○ Promptly identify suspect patients.

○ Utilize effective precautions in patients with suspected or proven tuberculosis.

○ Provide accurate useful information to family members of patients with tuberculosis.

Tuberculosis

I. Incidence of tuberculosis.
   A. TB has been declining throughout the century.
   B. National incidence is between 10 and 15 new cases each year per 100,000 population.
   C. Local variations include an incidence in excess of 50 per 100,000 in urban areas such as New York City and variable state incidences (approximately 20 per 100,000 in Florida).

II. Characteristics of organism.
   A. A rod-shaped bacterium *Mycobacterium tuberculosis*.
   B. Organism requires oxygen for growth.
   C. Organism extremely sensitive to ultraviolet light (sunshine); dies within a few hours when exposed to open air.
   D. Proteinaceous material and sputum may dry around coughed-up organisms and protect them. These can float in the air as droplet nuclei for hours.

III. Pathogenesis of disease.
   A. Droplet nuclei are sufficiently small to be inhaled into alveoli in lower lobe of the lung.
   B. Organism multiplies slowly, once every 14 to 24 hours.
   C. With inadequate host defenses, organism can enter lymphatics from the alveolus and travel to the hilar and mediastinal lymph nodes of the lungs.
   D. Some spill over into the circulatory system and travel to kidneys, bone, liver, brain, or lung apex.
   E. Most of the organisms spread through the blood and eventually settle in the apices of the lungs where the high oxygen concentration favors growth of the bacteria.
   F. Symptoms at this stage are of a mild bronchitis. If systemic spread is not controlled, miliary tuberculosis (multiple small infectious nodules throughout the body) results.

IV. Host response to TB.
   A. Certain lymphocytes, initially produced in the thymus and called T-lymphocytes, respond to the materials from the tubercle bacilli.
   B. T-lymphocytes release substances that cause inflammation around the tubercle bacilli and attract cells of the lung, called macrophages, which ingest the bacilli and try to kill them.

C. The immune response is usually sufficient to wall off primary infection before extensive damage.

D. Organisms survive in this walled off area (a granuloma) but are dormant.

E. This primary infection of the lower lobe and lymph node may calcify and show up on an X-ray as a Ghon complex.

V. Reactivation of tuberculosis.

A. When body's resistance falls, reactivation may occur, most often in lung apices.

B. Diseases or therapy that depresses lymphocyte/macrophage (cellular) immunity, such as steroids, lymphoma, Hodgkin's disease, results in reactivation.

C. Reactivation causes inflammation, cheese-like tissue necrosis (caseation), and cavities.

VI. Miliary and primary progressive tuberculosis.

A. Miliary tuberculosis is a widespread disease in which tubercle bacilli grow in many organs, causing tiny granulomas that resemble millet seeds. It is the commonest cause of tuberculous meningitis and pleuritis.

B. Primary progressive pulmonary tuberculosis is a lower-lobe bronchopneumonic disease in which the primary infection is not controlled and tissue necrosis with cavitation may occur.

VII. Signs and symptoms of reactivation tuberculosis—more than 90 percent of all active tuberculous cases are actually reactivations.

A. Usually no observable symptoms in the early stages.

B. By the time symptoms occur, disease is moderately or extensively progressive.

C. Common symptoms include cough, fever, night sweats, fatigue, weight loss, hoarseness, chest pain, and bloody sputum. Medical history is the key to diagnosis.

D. Patients with unsuspected reactivation tuberculosis are the principal source of new cases. Therefore, prevention of tuberculosis depends upon identification of all individuals with either active or dormant TB.

E. With reactivation, organisms generally involve the apices of the lungs where they cause extensive tissue destruction. When this necrosis of tissue reaches a bronchus, the material is coughed out, leaving behind a cavity in the lung (Figure 11-1, page 262).

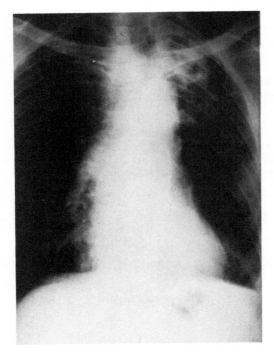

Figure 11-1: Chest X-ray of patient with cavitary tuberculosis, cavity in left apex.

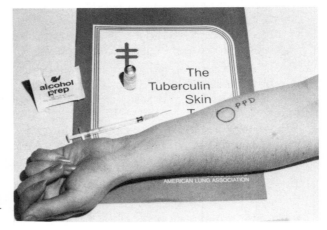

Figure 11-2: An intradermal PPD test.

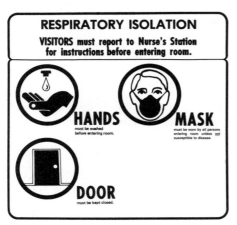

Figure 11-3: Respiratory isolation is used in cases of suspected or untreated tuberculosis. (Courtesy, St. Joseph's Hospital, Tampa.)

F. Spread through the bloodstream may occur with reactivation and result in secondary foci in meninges, bone, kidneys, brain, liver, lymph nodes, or the reproductive tract.

G. Extrapulmonary reactivation can occur at sites to which organisms spread during the primary infection. These patients, frequently without abnormal chest X-ray, may present with fever of unknown origin. The source of reactivation can be a bone focus, tuberculous meningitis, tuberculosis of the kidney, the adrenal gland, the ovaries, or a lymph node.

VIII. Diagnosis and prevention of tuberculosis.

A. Although chest X-ray has been used in the past, the PPD skin test (Figure 11-2), with material prepared from a culture of tuberculosis, is the most reliable way of detecting individuals who have or have had tuberculosis.

1. Material from the organism is called purified protein derivative (PPD). It is prepared from culture medium in which *M. tuberculosis* has grown.

2. A positive test indicates the presence of live bacilli in the body, active or dormant.

3. Skin testing methods include multiple-puncture and single-needle techniques. Multiple-puncture or "tine" tests are used as screening tools. The single-needle injection is more accurate.

4. From 48 to 72 hours after the injection, the size and type of reaction is evaluated by a trained individual.

5. No reaction or one smaller than 4 mm is considered negative.

6. A (reddened) raised area 5 to 9 mm is a questionable result and should be repeated.

7. A reaction of 10 mm or greater is evidence of past or present infection, a positive reaction.

8. Individuals not tested within four years may not give positive tests until they have had two tests within a month. This is referred to as stimulation of immune memory or the booster effect.

9. All close contacts of infectious patients should be immediately skin-tested. After eight weeks, they should again receive a skin test if initially negative. It should be repeated in eight to 10 weeks. If still negative, disease is ruled out.

10. Under certain circumstances of malnutrition, steroid therapy, widespread cancer, or immune deficiency, a false negative reaction may be obtained. In addition, other clinical states, such as smallpox, measles, and rubella vaccination, may cause a false negative.

11. All hospital employees should have an annual skin test. Those with frequent contact with tuberculous patients should be tested every six months. Repeated skin tests do not cause sensitization.

12. Size of reaction should always be recorded. A significant change from less than 10 mm to greater than 10 mm within two years constitutes a tuberculous conversion. One year of preventive TB chemotherapy is recommended for such converters to reduce number of surviving mycobacteria and insure that the disease is maximally walled off.

B. Preventive therapy—indications.

1. Preventive therapy for one year for PPD converters is recommended, consisting of daily isoniazid.

2. Preventive therapy for close contacts of an infectious individual should be continued through the eight weeks' follow-up. If then negative, stop chemotherapy. If positive, continue isoniazid for full year.

3. Individuals younger than 35 years of age with dormant tuberculosis (positive PPD) who have not previously received chemotherapy should be considered for one year of isoniazid.

4. Preventive therapy is indicated for individuals with dormant tuberculosis (PPD) who also have one or more of the following: alcoholism, diabetes, gastrostomy, corticosteroid therapy, silicosis, malignancy, sarcoidosis, lymphoma, X-ray therapy, cancer chemotherapy, or debility of old age.

C. Diagnostic studies.

1. Since positive skin test merely indicates presence of live but not necessarily invasive bacilli somewhere in the body, tests are required to detect active disease.

2. *M. tuberculosis* is rapidly identified by its staining properties. It retains carbolfuchsin or certain fluorescent stains despite washing with acid alcohol. Pink-stained organisms may be seen under the microscope, the fluorescent more easily under a fluorescence microscope.

a.) Single sputum specimens are collected in early morning on three consecutive days.

b.) Positive acid-fast smear is considered suggestive of active TB, since approximately 10,000/ml are needed to give a positive smear.

c.) Negative acid-fast smear does not rule out TB, since too few organisms may be present to be easily found under the microscope.

d.) A culture is more sensitive but requires three to six weeks to be completed.

e.) Cultured mycobacteria should be tested for specific antimicrobial sensitivities.

f.) A positive culture is diagnostic of active disease.

3. Isolation practices: Any patient admitted to the hospital with suspected or untreated tuberculosis is placed in respiratory isolation (Figure 11-3). Maintain until patient has had two weeks' effective therapy or three consecutive negative smears. Infected patients don't communicate TB unless their sputum contains enough bacteria to be smear-positive.

a.) Room requires rapid air exchange and exhaust to minimize droplet nuclei in the air.

b.) Emphasis is on good barrier technique: Patient covers nose and mouth with a tissue when coughing, sneezing, or laughing. Contaminated tissue is disposed of immediately in an impervious bag. Mask is worn by patient when outside the room and, ideally, whenever someone visits in the room. Masks are required for susceptible visitors. Visiting privileges are limited to immediate family and close friends, who have probably been exposed even before the patient's hospitalization. Good hand-washing technique required. No additional precautions are necessary.

c.) Once a positive smear is obtained, chemotherapy should be started within 48 hours to reduce the infectiousness of the patient.

d.) Isoniazid usually is in the regimen as well as one or more of a long list of antimicrobials. Combination of two or more drugs is usually recommended to minimize organisms developing drug resistance.

e.) As the patient responds, infectiousness rapidly decreases. After two weeks of intensive effective drug therapy, there is no need for further isolation.

f.) Patient may return home at any time in the treatment regimen that the clinical condition permits.

g.) Home isolation is unnecessary after three days of active treatment, since persons outside the hospital are not as compromised as patients inside, and those in the house may be presumed to have been exposed earlier.

h.) Patient with pulmonary TB can almost always be discharged before laboratory culture is reported.

i.) If smear-positive sputum is found from a patient not on respiratory isolation, a contact list of personnel and patients is necessary, since the patient is producing enough airborne organisms to infect others. If the smear is negative, but only the culture is positive, excretion of organisms into the air is assumed to be insignificant, and a contact list and follow-up are unnecessary.

4. Local health department must be notified of all cases of presumptive or proven tuberculosis. Many local health departments screen family and contacts, provide free drugs and follow-up.

5. Chemotherapy usually lasts 18 to 24 months. Shorter regimens, as short as six months, are under study. A nine-month regimen incorporating rifampin and isoniazid has been proven effective. Patients must be monitored for side effects of drugs.

6. With good patient compliance, therapy is 99 percent effective. Effectiveness is judged by clearing organisms from sputum, improvement in chest X-ray, weight gain, and reduced cough. Education should stress taking medications at the same time every day, to develop reliable habits.

7. Failure to respond is almost always due to failure of patient compliance.

IX. Risk of tuberculosis in hospital employees.

   A. One to two percent of hospital employees acquire the infection each year.

B. When the rate exceeds two percent, special precautions and more frequent testing of employees should be undertaken.

C. Disease acquisition is documented by PPD skin test conversion.

D. Most common source of TB for hospital employees is unsuspected patient.

    1. Patient thought to have cancer.

    2. Patient thought to have simple bacterial pneumonia.

    3. Patient with a cough and FUO.

E. Patient's specimens are handled in the laboratory under a bacteriologic hood to avoid exposure of the technician and contamination of the specimen. Several hours are required for processing. Acid-fast smears are usually available in 24 to 48 hours.

F. If a tuberculous patient is scheduled for other procedures, the appropriate department should be notified of the diagnosis. Nonemergency procedures should be postponed until the patient has had two weeks of chemotherapy. If surgery is essential, a totally disposable circuit should be used on anesthesia machines, and the machine carefully cleaned afterward, including changing the sodalime connector.

X. Drug therapy of TB.

A. Patients on therapy should be monitored carefully, since all the drugs have possible side effects.

B. Isoniazid, the usual drug, is given at an average dose of 300 mg daily. With more severe disease, higher doses may be used.

C. Ethambutol is a commonly used drug. Given in combination with isoniazid, the usual dose is 15 mg/kg per day.

D. With a high bacterial population, rifampin may be used in combination with isoniazid and ethambutol. The usual adult dosage is 600 mg a day. Principal toxicity is to the liver. The drug turns the urine red-orange; patient should be warned.

E. If laboratory sensitivity tests indicate the need for a change, alternative drugs may be used. Streptomycin, the most common, may be ototoxic. The drug should be avoided in patients with renal insufficiency.

F. Para-aminosalicylic acid (PAS) is a frequently used alternative drug. Liver and gastrointestinal side effects are possible.

G. In certain areas, free treatment and care are provided by the local health department.

Tuberculosis

XI. Nontuberculous mycobacterial infections.

A. A wide variety of nontuberculous mycobacteria, formerly called atypical or anonymous mycobacteria, can cause human infections. These organisms also give positive acid-fast smears, so such patients are frequently isolated early in the course as a precautionary measure. Among these mycobacteria are *M. kansasii, M. marinum, M. avium, M. intracellularis, M. fortuitum,* and *M. chelonei.*

B. Since person-to-person transmission is not a problem within the hospital, isolation is unnecessary once the organism is identified as nontuberculous. These organisms give negative niacin tests, whereas *M. tuberculosis* gives a positive.

C. Such diseases may or may not respond to the same drugs used with TB. Usually three to four drugs are employed. Others, such as erythromycin or the tetracyclines, may be tried.

T·E·S·T

---

1. The incidence of tuberculosis in the United States is
   a. declining.
   b. increasing.
   c. constant.
2. The highest incidence of tuberculosis in the United States occurs in
   a. poverty-stricken rural areas.
   b. cities and Indian reservations.
   c. the mountain states.
   d. white middle-class males.
3. Tuberculosis is transmitted by
   a. droplet nuclei.
   b. fomites.
   c. drinking water.
   d. contaminated food.
   e. contaminated hands.
4. Tuberculosis causes its initial infection most commonly in
   a. the upper lobes of the lungs.
   b. the lower lobes of the lungs.
   c. the skin.
   d. the bloodstream.
   e. the sinuses.
5. A positive TB skin test (PPD) always indicates
   a. active tuberculosis.
   b. presence of TB infection at some time in the person's life.
   c. infection at the site of the skin test.
6. The most important step in preventing spread of tuberculosis is
   a. trapping the patient's secretions and droplets in mask and tissues.
   b. wearing gloves and gown to protect against contamination.
   c. decontaminating all dishes and other utensils used in caring for the patient.

Answers are on page 270.

A·N·S·W·E·R·S

1. a. declining.
2. b. cities and Indian reservations.
3. a. droplet nuclei.
4. b. the lower lobes of the lungs.
5. b. presence of TB infection at some time in the person's life.
6. a. trapping the patient's secretions and droplets in mask and tissues.

12

Aspects of total parenteral nutrition

Purpose

Total parenteral nutrition (TPN) is being employed with increasing frequency for innumerable medical indications. The underlying medical conditions in recipients of TPN, the nature of the alimentation fluid itself, and the requirement for prolonged central venous catheterization predispose patients to many infectious complications. Prevention of such infections is a shared responsibility of physician, pharmacist, nurse, and patient alike. This section should acquaint nursing personnel with fundamental aspects of TPN, infection risks associated with various aspects of the practice, and appropriate preventive steps. A final section deals with diagnosis of infection in patients receiving TPN.

Learning objectives

○ State common indications for TPN.

○ Describe techniques for administering TPN.

○ List infectious complications of TPN.

○ Enumerate steps to reduce infectious complications of TPN.

○ Describe technique for diagnosis of infectious complications of TPN.

Total parenteral nutrition

Behavioral objectives

○ Identify candidate patients for TPN.

○ Utilize proper procedure in administration of TPN.

○ Employ proper procedure for specimen collection and identification of infection in TPN patients.

I. Indications for TPN.
   A. Severe acute or chronic malnutrition.
   B. Life-threatening malabsorption.
   C. Pre- or postsurgical state.
      1. Gastrointestinal obstruction.
      2. Ulcerative colitis.
      3. Pancreatitis.
      4. Diverticulitis.
      5. Gastrointestinal fistula.
      6. Congenital gastrointestinal anomalies.
      7. Crohn's disease.
      8. Burns.
      9. Chronic wound infections and decubitus ulcers.
      10. Extensive trauma.
      11. Short bowel syndrome.
   D. Medical illness complicated by malnutrition.
      1. Severe hypermetabolic states.
      2. Reversible coma.
      3. Malignant disease.
      4. Reversible liver disease.
      5. Acute and chronic renal failure.

II. Technique of TPN.
   A. Hyperosmolar solutions must be administered into a central vein (vena cava). Lipid emulsion can be given into a peripheral vein.
   B. IV line placed under strict aseptic circumstances.

C. TPN is generally given for prolonged periods, most exceeding one week.

D. Formula established according to individual patient needs.
   1. There are differences in adult and child calorie needs and trace metal/supplementary vitamin requirements.
   2. There is reduced nitrogen tolerance in hepatic and renal failure patients.
   3. Hypermetabolic state of burn patient requires added calories for protein sparing.

E. Lipid emulsion resolves two problems.
   1. Caloric requirements.
   2. Essential fatty acid requirements.

F. Typical daily adult TPN.
   1. Volume 2,500 to 4,000 ml.
   2. Carbohydrate calories 2,500 to 5,000.
   3. Lipid calories 500 to 1,000.
   4. Protein 100 to 150 grams.
   5. Electrolytes: sodium, potassium, magnesium, calcium, phosphate.
   6. Vitamins: vitamin A, D, E, C, thiamine, riboflavin, pyridoxine, niacin, pantothenic acid.

III. Complications of TPN.
   A. Infectious complications.
      1. Fungal infections predominate, accounting for more than 50 percent of infections in many institutions.
      2. Sepsis rate ranges from less than 7 percent to greater than 30 percent.
      3. Infections arise from IV puncture site, infusion fluid, underlying host disease sites.
   B. Metabolic complications—nutritional or therapeutic incompatibilities, excess, or deficiencies.
      1. Vitamin deficiencies or toxicities.
      2. Essential fatty acid deficiency.
      3. Trace metal deficiency.
      4. Glucose intolerance.
      5. Electrolyte and acid-base imbalance.
      6. Precipitation, binding, or inactivation of components.

Total parenteral nutrition

IV. Nursing practices to minimize infection complications.
    A. Assure strict asepsis in preparation of solutions.
        1. Central pharmacy preparation preferable, using laminar flow hood.
        2. Limit storage time of prepared solutions to less than 12 hours.
        3. Check solution for turbidity and particulate matter before administering.
    B. Catheter placement.
        1. Strict aseptic technique with gowns, masks, and gloves recommended.
        2. Defatting skin with acetone may increase infection rate.
        3. If possible, avoid placement near an active infection or heavily colonized site.
        4. Use effective antibacterial, such as iodophor.
        5. Place antibacterial ointment at puncture site.
        6. Cover with transparent air-permeable sterile dressing, leaving puncture site open (optional).
        7. Place occlusive dressing over transparent covering.
    C. IV catheter maintenance.
        1. Inspect every shift for leakage and local inflammation (do not remove dressing).
        2. Maintain an occlusive dressing.
        3. Change dressing every 48 to 72 hours with aseptic no-touch technique.
        4. Apply antibacterial at catheter site with each dressing change.
    D. Miscellaneous nursing considerations.
        1. No piggyback infusions or other medications through TPN line.
        2. No blood drawn from TPN line.
        3. In-line filter (0.22 micron) may be valuable; lipid solutions may be incompatible.
        4. If redness, tenderness, or purulent drainage appear at catheter site, catheter should be removed.
        5. TPN team may be of value in limiting sepsis incidence.
        6. Change administration tubing every 24 hours.

V. Diagnosis of sepsis in TPN recipient.
   A. Any fever should suggest sepsis.
   B. New occurrence of fever without obvious source is an indication for changing catheter site.
   C. Procedure to follow at first sign of fever.
      1. Discontinue infusion.
      2. Change infusion fluid and infusion line.
      3. Collect 5 ml fluid from infusion line for culture. Cleanse tubing with betadine, aspirate through 25-g needle into sterile syringe (or send tubing with cap on end to bacteriology).
      4. Collect 10 ml fluid from infusion bottle for culture.
      5. Inspect IV site.
      6. Culture any obvious purulent drainage from IV site.
      7. If catheter is to be changed, draw two blood cultures through the TPN catheter, cleanse around the catheter carefully with alcohol, remove the catheter aseptically, and culture the tip semiquantitatively and in a tube of culture broth.
      8. Collect two blood cultures from two different peripheral venous sites.

Total parenteral nutrition

T·E·S·T

1. True/False. Hyperosmolar solutions containing 20 percent glucose may be conveniently administered into an arm vein.
2. Which of the following is added to TPN solutions to both enhance caloric content and avoid essential-fatty-acid deficiencies?
   a. vitamins.   b. trace minerals.
   c. lipid emulsion.   d. amino acids.
3. Which is the predominant complication of TPN?
   a. hyperglycemia.   b. infection.
   c. fluid overload.   d. vitamin deficiency.
4. Ideally, prepared TPN solutions should be used within how many hours?
   a. 6.   b. 12.
   c. 24.   d. 48.
5. Which of the following can reduce infections in TPN?
   a. strict aseptic technique   b. prep the site with
   c. avoid placement near   an effective antibacterial.
      an active infection.   d. cover with an occlusive dressing.
   e. all of the above.
6. If fever develops in a patient receiving TPN, what should you suspect?
   a. drug fever.   b. urinary tract infection.
   c. IV sepsis.   d. factitious fever.

A·N·S·W·E·R·S

1. False. Solutions containing 20 percent glucose cause extreme pain and thrombosis of small veins. They must be given into large central veins.
2. c. lipid emulsion.
3. b. infection.
4. b. 12.
5. e. all of the answers, a–d.
6. c. IV sepsis.

Index

277

Index

278

Index

Index

Index

Index

Other titles of related interest from
MEDICAL ECONOMICS BOOKS

Manual for IV Therapy Procedures
Shila R. Channell, R.N., Ph.D.
ISBN 0-87489-238-4

Pediatric Policies, Procedures, and Personnel
Eileen M. Sporing, R.N., M.S.N., Mary K. Walton, R.N., M.S.N.,
and Charlotte C. Welch, R.N., M.S.N.
ISBN 0-87489-339-9

For information, write to:

MEDICAL ECONOMICS BOOKS
Oradell, New Jersey 07649
Or dial toll-free: 1-800-223-0581, ext. 2755
(Within the 201 area: 262-3030, ext. 2755)